D0999361

*Study Guide to
Accompany*

Advanced Pediatric Assessment

Ellen M. Chiocca, MSN, CPNP, APN, RNC-NIC, is a clinical assistant professor in the School of Nursing at DePaul University. She received a master of science degree in nursing and a postmaster nurse practitioner certificate from Loyola University, Chicago, and a bachelor of science degree in nursing from St. Xavier University. Prior to joining the faculty at DePaul University, she taught at Loyola University, Chicago, from 1991 to 2013. Ms. Chiocca's clinical specialty is the nursing of children. Her research focuses on how various forms of violence affect children's health. She is certified in neonatal intensive care nursing and as a pediatric nurse practitioner. In addition to teaching at DePaul, Ms. Chiocca also continues clinical practice as a pediatric nurse practitioner at a community clinic in Chicago. Ms. Chiocca has published more than 25 journal articles and book chapters, and is also a peer reviewer for the journal *Neonatal Network*. She is currently pursuing a PhD in nursing.

Study Guide to Accompany

Advanced Pediatric Assessment, Second Edition

A Case Study and Critical Thinking Review

Ellen M. Chiocca, MSN, CPNP, APN, RNC-NIC

SPRINGER PUBLISHING COMPANY

NEW YORK

Copyright © 2015 Springer Publishing Company, LLC

All rights reserved.

No part of this publication may be reproduced, stored in a retrieval system, or transmitted in any form or by any means, electronic, mechanical, photocopying, recording, or otherwise, without the prior permission of Springer Publishing Company, LLC, or authorization through payment of the appropriate fees to the Copyright Clearance Center, Inc., 222 Rosewood Drive, Danvers, MA 01923, 978-750-8400, fax 978-646-8600, info@copyright.com or on the Web at www.copyright.com.

Springer Publishing Company, LLC
11 West 42nd Street
New York, NY 10036
www.springerpub.com

Acquisitions Editor: Elizabeth Nieginski
Composition: diacriTech

ISBN: 978-0-8261-6177-2
e-book ISBN: 978-0-8261-6178-9
ISBN (Textbook): 978-0-8261-6175-8
e-book ISBN (Textbook): 978-0-8261-6176-5
Set ISBN: 978-0-8261-2862-1
Set e-book ISBN: 978-0-8261-2868-3

14 15 16 17 / 5 4 3 2 1

The author and the publisher of this Work have made every effort to use sources believed to be reliable to provide information that is accurate and compatible with the standards generally accepted at the time of publication. Because medical science is continually advancing, our knowledge base continues to expand. Therefore, as new information becomes available, changes in procedures become necessary. We recommend that the reader always consult current research and specific institutional policies before performing any clinical procedure. The author and publisher shall not be liable for any special, consequential, or exemplary damages resulting, in whole or in part, from the readers' use of, or reliance on, the information contained in this book. The publisher has no responsibility for the persistence or accuracy of URLs for external or third-party Internet websites referred to in this publication and does not guarantee that any content on such websites is, or will remain, accurate or appropriate.

Library of Congress Cataloging-in-Publication Data
Chiocca, Ellen M.
  Study guide to accompany advanced pediatric assessment / Ellen M. Chiocca, MSN, CPNP, APN, RNC-NIC, assistant professor of clinical nursing, DePaul University, Chicago, Illinois, pediatric nurse practitioner, Heartland Health Outreach, Chicago, Illinois.
      pages cm
  Includes bibliographical references.
  ISBN 978-0-8261-6177-2
  1. Children—Medical examinations. 2. Children—Diseases—Diagnosis—Examinations, questions, etc.
I. Chiocca, Ellen M. Advanced pediatric assessment. II. Title.
  RJ50.C487 2015 Suppl.
  618.92'0075—dc23
                         2014035016

Special discounts on bulk quantities of our books are available to corporations, professional associations, pharmaceutical companies, health care organizations, and other qualifying groups. If you are interested in a custom book, including chapters from more than one of our titles, we can provide that service as well.

For details, please contact:
Special Sales Department, Springer Publishing Company, LLC
11 West 42nd Street, 15th Floor, New York, NY 10036-8002
Phone: 877-687-7476 or 212-431-4370; Fax: 212-941-7842
E-mail: sales@springerpub.com

Printed in the United States of America by McNaughton & Gunn.

I would like to dedicate this book to the memory of two great women—Barbara Chiocca Fogarty (1940–1989) and Ellen Mitchell Gaughan (1943–1975). My aunts, one paternal, one maternal. Each was the first woman on one side of the family to earn a college degree. Both women loved school, learning, and books. Both women encouraged me to achieve in school. I think about both of my aunts frequently, and I miss them. I know that a little part of each of them lives on in me. And to Bella and Ralph, always.

Contents

Preface

The purpose of the *Study Guide to Accompany Advanced Pediatric Assessment, Second Edition: A Case Study and Critical Thinking Review* is to assist the student or novice pediatric health care provider in solidifying the specialized knowledge and skills that are required when conducting a pediatric history and physical examination. Each chapter of this *Study Guide* aligns with the corresponding textbook chapter. The chapters in this book follow a uniform format, presenting a chapter overview, expected learning outcomes for the chapter, essential terminology, and critical thinking exercises in two formats: short-answer, and case study. The chapters continue with certification exam–style, multiple-choice questions (with answers), and sample documentation to show examples of subjective and objective findings that are necessary to record.

It is important for all health care providers to be sure that children receive the highest quality care possible at a time when their young bodies and minds are growing and developing. It is my hope that this *Study Guide* will help to augment the student's learning, and increase the learner's confidence in providing comprehensive, high-quality care to children of all ages.

Ellen M. Chiocca

Acknowledgments

I would like to thank Elizabeth Nieginski, executive editor at Springer Publishing Company, who helped me bring the idea of this *Study Guide* to life. She was very open to and enthusiastic about my ideas, and always encouraging along the way.

I must acknowledge the beautiful, innocent, and loving children that I have had the honor and privilege to care for in my 32 years as a pediatric nurse.

And thank you, of course, to Ralph and Isabella, for everything.

Child Health Assessment: An Overview

CHAPTER OVERVIEW

Health assessment of infants, children, and adolescents requires specialized knowledge and skills. Rapid anatomic, physiologic, developmental, and psychosocial changes occur from the moment and infant is born, and continue through adolescence. These changes affect how the pediatric health care provider must approach the health care encounter, including how to communicate with the child and family, what historical information to obtain, how to conduct the physical examination, and in what sequence. Because of a child's physical and psychological immaturity, the child as patient is never viewed in isolation, but as part of the parent–child dyad, family, and community.

Expected Learning Outcomes

After reading Chiocca, *Advanced Pediatric Assessment, Second Edition*, Chapter 1, the learner will be able to:

1. Understand the anatomic and physiologic differences that exist between infants, children, and adults
2. Explain the potential clinical implications of multiple body system immaturity in the pediatric patient
3. Explain why the health care provider's approach to the pediatric history and physical examination changes with the child's age and developmental level
4. Discuss how a child's developmental level affects the health care provider's approach to communication with the child and caregiver
5. Discuss the parent–child relationship in the context of the pediatric health care encounter

Essential Terminology

Absorption—in pharmacokinetics, the movement of a drug from its entry site into the bloodstream

Alveoli—small, balloon-like structures in the lung where gas exchange takes place

Apocrine gland—a type of sweat gland; does not become active until puberty

Blood–brain barrier—the semipermeable membrane that protects the brain from toxins and harmful substances in the blood

Cell-mediated immunity—a type of acquired immunity mediated predominantly by T lymphocyte cells

Cephalocaudal—head to toe

Distribution—in pharmacokinetics, the movement of a drug throughout the bloodstream

Eccrine gland—a type of sweat gland

Epidermis—the outermost, avascular layer of the skin

Esotropia—inward deviation of the eye

Eustachian tube—the structure that connects the middle ear to the nasopharynx

Excretion—in pharmacokinetics, the process of removing drug metabolites from the body, usually through the urine or stool

Humoral immunity—a type of acquired immunity mediated predominantly by circulating antibodies

Innocent murmur—nonpathologic heart murmur

Lordosis—convex curvature of the spine

Menarche—the first menstrual period

Metabolism—in pharmacokinetics, the breakdown of a drug that occurs in the liver

Milia—epidermal cysts in neonates caused by the accumulation of sebum

Myelination—the formation of the myelin sheath around a nerve, which permits nerve impulses to move more quickly

Nystagmus—rapid involuntary movements of the eyes

Passive immunity—immunity produced by the transfer to one person of antibodies that were produced by another person

Pinna—the visible part of the ear seen outside the head

Proximodistal—near to far; for example, shoulder to fingertips

Stratum corneum—the outermost layer of the epidermis

Thelarche—the onset of breast development in girls; heralds the onset of puberty

CRITICAL THINKING EXERCISES

Short-Answer Critical Thinking Exercises

1. What is meant by the phrase, "children are not just little adults"? Be specific and give examples.
2. Name the six age groups that are discussed in *Advanced Pediatric Assessment, Second Edition*, and specify the corresponding age parameters for each.
3. For each body system or function listed in Table 1.1 of the *Advanced Pediatric Assessment, Second Edition* textbook, name and discuss at least three clinical implications of anatomic and physiologic immaturity.
4. What are the clinical implications of young children having a greater body surface area than adults?

5. Neonates and infants have reduced catecholamine stores. How does this affect their response to a hypotensive event?

6. Discuss the pharmacologic implications of body system immaturity in the pediatric patient.

Critical Thinking Case Study Exercises

Exercise 1

Cara is a 2-month-old infant who has been brought to the clinic by her mother for a well-infant exam. Her mother states that she has been using powdered formula for Cara, but the cost has become an issue because her husband lost his job, so she has been diluting the formula slightly more than the manufacturer's directions dictate. In addition, Cara's mother states that since it is summer, she has been sure to give Cara extra Nursery Water when the weather is hot and humid, because their home lacks air conditioning in their home.

1. Is slight dilution of infant formula harmful to an infant this age? Why or why not?
2. Does the administration of extra Nursery Water affect Cara in any way? If so, how?
3. Which body system is it important to think about in this situation?

Exercise 2

Patrick is a 10-month-old who was brought to the urgent care center by his father. Patrick has been running a low-grade fever for approximately 2 days, with copious green nasal secretions. He is alert, happy, and playful during the exam, but upon auscultation of the chest, crackles are heard bilaterally. The provider uses a bulb syringe to remove all nasal secretions, and auscultates Patrick's chest again. Despite the fact that Patrick is now crying and much less cooperative, his lungs are clear.

1. Explain how the presence of nasal secretions affects the assessment of breath sounds in a child this age.
2. Does the presence of nasal secretions from Patrick's nose have anything to do with his breath sounds? If yes, explain.
3. Is Patrick still an obligate nose breather?

Exercise 3

Jeremiah is a 4-month-old who is brought to the clinic by his mother for a health maintenance exam. He was born at 37-weeks gestation after his mother began premature labor due to a urinary tract infection. There were no perinatal complications and Jeremiah went home with his mother after 48 hours. Jeremiah is being exclusively breastfed and has not received any solid food. Today, his mother has several concerns: (a) that Jeremiah is unable to hear, (b) that he may be anemic, and (c) that his left eye turns inward at intervals.

1. What primitive reflex could be elicited to assess Jeremiah's hearing? Is that reflex still present in an infant this age?
2. Should blood be drawn to assess for anemia? Why or why not?
3. Does Jeremiah need an ophthalmology referral? Why or why not?

Exercise 4

Tina, aged 15 years, comes to the school-based health center with moderate dysmenorrhea. As she watches the health care provider complete documentation, Tina notices health posters on the clinic wall that prompt her to ask questions about things she has read on the Internet and learned in health class. She asks the following:

1. How does one know when puberty starts and what happens first?
2. What causes acne to start in adolescence?
3. What causes body odor to start in adolescence?
4. What does it mean that the brain is not fully mature until late adolescence?

REVIEW QUESTIONS

1. Neonates are more prone to respiratory conditions than older infants, children, and adults. One reason for this is that the number of alveoli present in the term infant is:

   a. Ten percent of the total number of alveoli found in the adult lung
   b. Fifteen percent of the total number of alveoli found in the adult lung
   c. Twenty-five percent of the total number of alveoli found in the adult lung
   d. Fifty percent of the total number of alveoli found in the adult lung

2. Which of the following anatomic or physiologic differences in the respiratory tract exists in young children?

   a. Proportionately smaller epiglottis
   b. Larynx is located two to three cervical vertebrae lower
   c. Proportionately smaller soft palate
   d. Diaphragmatic breathing until approximately age 6 years

3. The trachea is proportionately shorter and smaller in diameter in young children. The clinical implications of this include all of the following *except*:

   a. Greater potential for airway obstruction
   b. Decreased resistance to airflow
   c. Inhaled air is warmed and humidified less effectively
   d. The risk of aspiration is increased

4. Infants and toddlers are more prone to middle ear infections and effusions because their:

   a. Eustachian tubes are short and straight
   b. Eustachian tubes lie in a relatively vertical plane
   c. External auditory canal is short and straight
   d. External auditory canal is straight with an upward curve

5. The younger the child, the more rapid the heart rate because of:

   a. Low body weight
   b. Low oxygen demands
   c. High oxygen demands
   d. High blood pressure

6. Infants are more prone to hypothermia because of which of the following?

   a. Increased body surface area
   b. Proportionately smaller head
   c. Overdeveloped sweating and vasoconstriction mechanisms
   d. Moderately high amounts of subcutaneous fat

7. Renal function, including the glomerular filtration rate, is immature until age:

   a. 1 year
   b. 2 years
   c. 3 years
   d. 5 years

8. When prescribing oral medications to a 4-month-old, the pediatric health care provider must consider which of the following?

   a. Pancreatic enzyme activity is decreased until approximately age 4 to 6 months; this may affect bioavailability of certain drugs
   b. Gastric pH is acidotic, affecting oral medication absorption
   c. Hepatic enzyme activity is decreased until approximately age 3 to 4 years; this speeds up drug metabolism in children
   d. Infants and young children have a rapid gastric emptying time, affecting the rate of drug absorption

9. Care must be taken when prescribing topical medications to infants and children younger than age 2 years because:

   a. Infants and young children are more likely to rub off the medication
   b. A thin epidermis results in more rapid absorption of drugs
   c. Topical medications are not effective in this age group; the equivalent oral form of the drug must be prescribed
   d. It is too difficult to titrate a safe dose in this age group

10. Infants are more prone to increased body temperature and febrile seizures because of:

    a. Overdeveloped peripheral vasodilation mechanisms
    b. Underdeveloped peripheral vasodilation mechanisms
    c. Increased flushing when crying
    d. Decreased body surface area

11. The length of a young child's small intestine is larger with a greater surface area relative to body size. This results in:

    a. Less water absorption
    b. More water absorption
    c. Less electrolyte loss with liquid stools
    d. Firmer stools

12. The respiratory rate lowers to near adult levels around age 8 to 10 years because:

    a. Respirations become thoracic
    b. Cardiac function improves
    c. Less respiratory secretions are produced
    d. Tidal volume increases

13. Children have a higher metabolic rate than adults. Because of this, children are more prone to:

    a. Wound infection
    b. Weight gain
    c. Growth delay
    d. Dehydration

14. A child's radial pulse may not be easily palpable until age 6 years because of:

    a. Undeveloped left ventricular muscle
    b. High resting cardiac output
    c. Low systolic blood pressure
    d. Displaced apical impulse

15. Rib fractures are uncommon in young children because:

    a. The ribs do not protrude from the thorax
    b. The ribs are inflexible in young children
    c. The percentage of cartilage in ribs is high
    d. The normally protruding abdomen protects the ribs

16. Transient esotropia is within normal limits until age:

    a. 3 months
    b. 6 months
    c. 9 months
    d. 12 months

17. Infants and children metabolize drugs more slowly than adults because of:

    a. Low serum bilirubin concentrations
    b. Impaired liver conjugation reactions
    c. Higher levels of plasma albumin and globulin
    d. Decreased hepatic enzyme function

18. Which of the following is a clinical implication of an immature neurologic system in children?

    a. Beginning control of bowel and bladder does not occur until about age 2 years
    b. Neonates and very young infants have a less permeable blood–brain barrier, preventing the passage of large, lipid-soluble molecules
    c. The blood pressure is more consistent in the neonatal period
    d. Gross motor development occurs more slowly than fine motor development

19. Infectious illnesses are common in children aged 6 years and younger because of:

    a. An active reticuloendothelial system
    b. Underdeveloped cell-mediated and humoral immunity
    c. Higher amounts of fetal hemoglobin at birth
    d. Continued passive immunity after age 6 months

20. Young children have well-developed lymph tissue at birth and it continues to grow beyond normal adult size. At what age does lymph tissue begin to decrease to normal adult size?

    a. 6 to 8 years
    b. 8 to 10 years
    c. 10 to 12 years
    d. 12 to 14 years

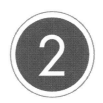

Assessment of Child Development and Behavior

CHAPTER OVERVIEW

The developmental assessment is an essential part of the health care of children of all ages. The child's age, health history, current developmental status, and reason for the health care visit dictate the type and depth of the developmental assessment. The pediatric health care provider must be proficient in identifying major developmental milestones in all developmental domains, be able to recognize signs that herald a developmental abnormality, and know when to conduct a developmental evaluation using standardized developmental screening tools.

Expected Learning Outcomes

After reading Chiocca, *Advanced Pediatric Assessment, Second Edition,* Chapter 2, the learner will be able to:

1. Identify normal physical and psychosocial growth and development in infants, children, and adolescents
2. Recognize deviations from normal physical and psychosocial growth and development in infants, children, and adolescents
3. Perform developmental assessments on children of various ages

Essential Terminology

Abstract thinking—conceptual thinking; understanding that words and concepts can have multiple meanings; develops in late school age–early adolescence

Cephalocaudal development—motor development that progresses in a head-to-toe direction

Cognitive development—development involving intellectual and adaptive skills

Concrete thinking—literal thinking; decision making, understanding, and processing is centered on the here and now

Critical sensitive period—developmental periods in which a child is particularly sensitive to developmental stimuli

Deductive reasoning—the process of reasoning from the general to the specific

Developmental evaluation—an in-depth developmental assessment using a standardized developmental screening tool

Developmental screening—a developmental examination using a standardized screening checklist; can be conducted by the health care provider or by parent report

Developmental surveillance—the ongoing process of monitoring a child's growth and development within the context of all health care encounters

Fine motor development—physical development involving the use of small muscles

Gross motor development—physical development involving the use of large muscles

Inductive reasoning—the process of reasoning from the specific to the general

Language development—the process by which children learn to communicate with sounds, gestures, and words; includes both expressive and receptive language abilities

Object permanence—the understanding that even if an object is not able to be detected with any senses, (for example, visible, tangible), it still exists

Proximodistal development—motor development that progresses in a near-to-far manner

Socioemotional development—psychosocial development of a child; encompasses behavior, temperament, parent–child interaction, peer and teacher interactions, school performance, and psychosocial development

Temperament—individual personality characteristics and behaviors

CRITICAL THINKING EXERCISES

Short-Answer Critical Thinking Exercises

1. Discuss the effect of temperament on an infant's or child's growth and development.
2. Discuss how an infant or child's situation can affect his or her growth and development.
3. Name some screening tools commonly used to assess developmental milestones in children, and compare and contrast them.
4. Why is developmental assessment essential in every pediatric health care visit?
5. Explain the differences between developmental surveillance, developmental screening, and developmental evaluation and for each, give an example of when and how to conduct the assessment.
6. Discuss how maternal depression affects child development for each developmental stage, from infancy through adolescence. What developmental domains are affected for each age group? Explain how and why each age group is affected differently by maternal depression.
7. Discuss why the prenatal, perinatal, and neonatal histories contain essential information when assessing a child with a developmental delay. What specific areas of each of these histories are important to focus on when evaluating motor, language, cognitive, and personal–social delays?

8. When conducting a developmental assessment on a child who is a new immigrant or refugee, what factors must the health care provider consider that may increase the child's risk for developmental delays?
9. What specific assessments are important to make?
10. Do the circumstances regarding the child's immigration affect the type and depth of developmental assessments? Why or why not?

Critical Thinking Case Study Exercises

Exercise 1

A 14-year-old African American girl, Tanya, presents to the clinic for a school physical. She is accompanied by her mother. Tanya is the oldest child in a two-parent home. She has two younger sisters, aged 12 and 10 years; her mother reports some sibling rivalry. Tanya is an "A/B" student with an occasional "C" grade. She is on the math team at school is very successful at this activity. During the health care encounter, Tanya is sullen and answers questions with one-word answers. She is testy and short-tempered with her mother. When her mother is out of the room during the sensitive part of the history, Tanya is less testy and opens up more with the health care provider. Her mother is concerned and asks if this behavior is normal and if her daughter needs help.

1. What other parts of Tanya's history are important to know?
2. Is Tanya's behavior within normal limits or a sign of a developmental or psychosocial concern?
3. What risk factors and protective factors exist for Tanya?
4. What should the health care provider conclude?

Exercise 2

Michael is a 12-month-old European American boy who is at the clinic for his annual health maintenance examination. He is accompanied by his mother and his 3-year-old sister. His biologic father is not involved. This is Michael's first time at this clinic; he does not have a medical home. He was born at 36 weeks gestation to a 22-year-old G_2P_2 mother who smoked cigarettes during her pregnancy. Michael's birth weight was 4 pounds (1.82 kg), his birth length was 19 inches (48.3 cm), and his head circumference was 13 inches (33 cm). The health care provider asks Michael's mother to fill out an Ages and Stages Questionnaire for a 12-month-old. This developmental assessment reveals the following:

Communication: Smiles, laughs; says baba, mama; does not play peek-a-boo (mother has never tried); follows simple commands sporadically

Gross motor: Does not take simple steps with hands being held; crawls well; is not pulling to stand

Fine motor: "Puts everything in his mouth"; uses all fingers and thumb to grasp items before picking them up

Problem solving: Looks for objects that are hidden; imitates behavior

Personal–social: Hugs a stuffed animal; beginning to know what to do when dressing in simple clothing

1. What other historical and physical assessments are important to obtain?
2. Is Michael's developmental assessment within normal limits? Why or why not?
3. What risk factors, if any, exist in Michael's medical history that would predispose him to developmental delays?
4. Are there any risk factors in Michael's social history that would predispose him to developmental delays?

Exercise 3

The expressive language assessment of an 18-month-old boy reveals that he speaks only three words with meaning. All other developmental assessments are within normal limits and his hearing is normal. His family speaks Arabic in the home and he attends day care for 8 hours a day, 5 days a week where the caregivers and other children speak English.

1. Explain how exposure to two languages at this developmental stage can affect his expressive language abilities.
2. Given his social history, is his language assessment considered within normal limits? Why or why not?

REVIEW QUESTIONS

1. The health care provider is performing a developmental assessment on a 4-month-old infant. The provider expects to observe which of the following gross motor abilities?

   a. Sits steadily without support
   b. Rolls from abdomen to back
   c. Rolls from back to abdomen
   d. Lifts chest and abdomen off flat surface

2. Which of the following primitive reflexes would be considered an *abnormal* finding at age 6 months?

   a. Babinski
   b. Extrusion
   c. Landau
   d. Corneal

3. Which of the following is a gross motor developmental red flag if observed in a 12-month-old child?

   a. Cannot walk independently
   b. Cannot crawl upstairs
   c. Cannot balance on one foot for one second
   d. Cannot bear weight when pulled to stand

4. A child who can walk down stairs using alternate footing, catch a bounced ball, and balance on one foot for 3 to 5 seconds would also be expected to:

   a. Draw a person with three parts
   b. Use scissors well

   c. Copy a diamond

   d. Tie shoelaces

5. Normal developmental milestones for a healthy 6-month-old infant include all of the following *except*:

   a. Presence of the Moro reflex

   b. Lifts head when prone

   c. Makes babbling noises

   d. Social smile

6. The mother of a 15-month-old toddler is concerned because her child frequently has tantrums when asked to share his toys. This behavior:

   a. Is normal and reflects ritualism

   b. Is normal and reflects egocentricity

   c. Is abnormal and is a sign of a behavior disorder

   d. Is abnormal and is a sign of separation anxiety

7. Cognitive development can best be evaluated in a 6-month-old infant by assessing:

   a. Head control

   b. Receptive language

   c. Object permanence

   d. Fine motor ability

8. A supine infant, when pulled to sit, should no longer have head lag by:

   a. 1 month

   b. 2 months

   c. 4 months

   d. 6 months

9. Which of the following is *always* a developmental red flag?

   a. Incorrect pronoun use

   b. Difficulty sharing

   c. Speech less than 75% unintelligible

   d. Loss of milestones

10. A major developmental task for the school-aged child is to:

   a. Separate from peers

   b. Question authority

   c. Master abstract thinking

   d. Separate from parents

11. A developmentally normal 5-year-old child should be able to draw a picture of a person with:

   a. 1 to 2 parts

   b. 2 to 4 parts

   c. 3 to 6 parts

   d. 6 to 8 parts

12. Which of the following describes normal expressive language abilities in an 18-month-old child?

    a. Says first word with meaning besides "mama," "dada," "baba"; imitates vocalizations; points to "ask" for something
    b. Approximately five-word vocabulary; understands simple commands; points to "ask" for something
    c. Approximately 20-word vocabulary; uses two-word phrases; 25% intelligibility; understands approximately 50 words
    d. Approximately 75-word vocabulary; uses two- to three-word phrases; 75% intelligibility; understands approximately 150 words

13. Which of the following descriptions of cognitive development during toddlerhood is accurate?

    a. Beginning abstract thinking
    b. Egocentrism
    c. Identifying more with peers
    d. Increased separation from parents

14. When performing a developmental examination on a 15-month-old toddler, which of the following is *not* a developmental task that needs to be considered?

    a. Stranger anxiety
    b. Negativism
    c. Separation anxiety
    d. Identity

15. Which of the following phrases as uttered by a toddler best describes the developmental "tone" of preschoolers?

    a. "I'll do it myself!"
    b. "Show me how."
    c. "I want to be alone."
    d. "Why?"

16. When using a standardized developmental assessment tool, all of the following must be considered *except*:

    a. The reliability and validity of the developmental assessment tool
    b. The sensitivity and specificity of the developmental assessment tool
    c. The language(s) in which the developmental assessment tool is available
    d. Whether the child lives in a single-parent household

17. Which of the following is an example of a developmental milestone that is within normal limits?

    a. A 15-month-old who pulls to stand but does not walk independently
    b. A 1-year-old who speaks two words besides "mama" and "dada"
    c. A 5-month-old with head lag
    d. A 2-year-old with a vocabulary of approximately 10 to 15 words

18. A child whose fine motor abilities include turning book pages one at a time, building a tower of six cubes, dressing herself in simple clothing, and imitating vertical or circular strokes when drawing is likely aged:

    a. 12 months
    b. 15 months
    c. 18 months
    d. 24 months

19. By 3 years of age, a normal, healthy child's expressive language abilities should be:

    a. Approximately 25% intelligible, using 20 or more words and two-word phrases
    b. Approximately 50% intelligible, using 50 or more words and two- to three-word phrases
    c. Approximately 75% intelligible, using at least 900 words and three- to four-word sentences
    d. Fully intelligible, using at least 1,500 words and complete sentences with use of past and future tense

20. A child's speech should be 100% intelligible by what age?

    a. 2 years
    b. 3 years
    c. 4 years
    d. 5 years

SAMPLE DOCUMENTATION

Patient Name _____ Date of Birth _____ Date _____
Gender_____

I. **Health History**
   A. **Reason for Seeking Health Care**
   B. **Past Medical History**
      1. Prenatal, birth, neonatal history (for example, prematurity, prolonged ventilation, ECMO)
      2. Injuries (type and severity, mechanism of injury)
      3. Emergency room visits (dates and reason for visit)
      4. Chronic conditions
      5. Past hospitalizations
      6. Surgical history
      7. Family medical history
      8. Current medications
         a. Prescription
         b. Over the counter
         c. Include exact dose, frequency, time of last dose given, reason for medication
      9. Alternative therapies used

      10. Immunization status (note delays)

      11. Review of systems

   C. Nutritional History

      1. Meal schedule

      2. 24-hour food intake for the past 3 to 5 days

      3. Bottle propping

      4. Appetite

      5. Voracious appetite

      6. Vomiting/rumination

      7. Dental visits

   D. Developmental History

      1. Milestones reached

      2. Behavior

      3. Temperament

      4. Prolonged screen time

   E. Sleep History

      1. Hours per day

      2. Difficulty sleeping/insomnia/hypersomnia

      3. Nightmares

   F. Social History

      1. Maternal support systems

      2. Family stresses/crises

      3. Parental mental illness or addiction

      4. Poor parental bonding

      5. Inappropriate dress for weather

      6. Teenage parents

      7. Parental knowledge deficits

      8. Poverty/homelessness

      9. School performance

      10. Behavior at school

      11. Truancy

      12. Frequent school tardiness

II. History of Present Illness (Development Complaint)

III. Physical Examination

   A. Vital Signs

   B. Anthropometric Measurements

      1. Weight

      2. Length/height

      3. Head circumference (age 3 years and younger)

      4. Weight for length/height (both height and weight below 5th percentile occur with longstanding neglect)

      5. Body mass index (age 2 years and older)

      6. Plot all measurements on growth charts

   C. Behavioral Assessment for Age

      1. Mood

      2. Affect

      3. Behavior

      4. Parent–child interaction

      5. Eye contact
      6. Smiling/interaction
      7. Presence/absence of stranger anxiety (infants/toddlers)
      8. Anxiety
      9. Agitation
    10. Apathy
    11. Dislikes being touched/held
    12. Preference of inanimate objects over toys or social interaction
    13. Irritability
    14. Lethargy

D. Developmental Assessment
      1. Objective developmental assessment for age (use formal developmental assessment tool)
      2. Temperament

E. Neurologic Assessment

F. Nutritional Assessment
      1. Tooth decay
      2. Skin turgor
      3. Note emaciated or malnourished appearance
      4. Overweight/obesity
      5. Alteration in elimination patterns

DEVELOPMENTAL/BEHAVIORAL ASSESSMENT: WRITE-UP

Use the space provided here to document all subjective and objective findings using the SOAP rubric.

Subjective—(historical information; chief complaint; medical and psychiatric co-morbidities)

Objective—(vital signs, physical examination findings, results of laboratory and other diagnostic tests; results of screening instruments)

Assessment—(diagnosis [use ICD-10 codes]; other health issues that are identified)

Plan—(treatment, medications, therapies, teaching, referrals, follow-up care)

Communicating With Children and Families

CHAPTER OVERVIEW

Effective communication is essential to building trusting relationships with pediatric patients and their families. The communication process with children can be complicated by physical, emotional, or cognitive impairment and needs to be targeted toward their developmental stage. The incorporation of the family is especially important when the patient is a child. Providers of care must understand the communication process and develop age-appropriate communication skills to administer patient-centered care.

Expected Learning Outcomes

After reading Chiocca, *Advanced Pediatric Assessment, Second Edition*, Chapter 3, the learner will be able to:

1. Describe the role and importance of the family in the patient care process
2. Identify and explain the elements of the communication process
3. Describe the differences in communication that characterize children at different developmental stages
4. Explain the various communication techniques and identify age groups for which they are appropriate

Essential Terminology

Active listening—the receiver objectively observes both the verbal and nonverbal aspects of the sender's message

Attentive listening—the receiver focuses on what the person is saying but actively compares the sender's experience with his or her own (Rider, 2011)

Avoidance language—the speaker uses word choices that avoid describing what he or she is trying to communicate, such as when a person is avoiding strong emotions and feelings about a subject (Hockenberry, 2011)

Communication—a process in which thoughts, ideas, feelings, messages, or information are exchanged through speech and nonverbal means such as behavior, body language, or eye contact

Distancing language—the use of impersonal language such as "it" or "others" to discuss situations pertaining to oneself or one's child (Hockenberry, 2011)

Empathy—the ability to understand and identify with another person's feelings

Involuntary body language—movements such as facial expressions that are usually provoked by emotion

Nonverbal communication—the sending and receiving of wordless messages, including body language, facial expressions, eye contact, clothing, hairstyles, and tone of voice and other qualities of speech (Stein, 2006)

Paralanguage—the vocal elements used to communicate, such as pitch, rate, inflection, volume, quality, enunciation, flatness, and fullness (Eisenberg, 2012)

Pretend listening—the receiver merely gives the appearance of listening

Selective listening—the receiver hears only what interests him or her, thereby missing important details

Sympathy—to share similar feelings with another person

Verbal communication—actual words, either spoken or written, that people use to communicate

Voluntary body language—intentional gestures and movements

CRITICAL THINKING EXERCISES

Short-Answer Critical Thinking Exercises

1. Discuss the communication process with someone. What are the roles each of you play in the process? What are the elements that influence the process?
2. Describe nonverbal communication that could be viewed as negative.
3. Provide three pediatric-specific issues that can affect communication.
4. Discuss the differences in the communication process when talking with children of different developmental ages.
5. Discuss how culture, past experience, and emotional state can affect communication.
6. Discuss the importance of building rapport, especially with an adolescent. Provide three examples of how it can be done.
7. Describe why it is vital to use clear, concise language with young children.
8. Provide two options for communicating with a child who speaks English but has a parent who does not.
9. What is the role of play in communicating with children?
10. Describe three barriers to communication and give examples of methods to overcome them.
11. Discuss the elements of family dynamics on the communication process.

Critical Thinking Case Study Exercises

Exercise 1

Sara is an 18-month-old toddler who presents to the clinic with her mother because of a rash on her lower left leg. Her mother reports the rash has been there for 2 days but does not seem to be changing. Young toddlers speak approximately 10 to 15 words but their receptive speech is much greater.

1. Should you begin speaking with Sara or the mother first? Why?
2. How should you begin the exam?
3. What is the best method to use in approaching Sara?
4. How should directions be given to Sara?
5. You need to use special equipment to look at the rash. How do you explain this to Sara?

Exercise 2

José is a 6-year-old boy who is in the emergency department of the hospital for the first time in his life for suspected acute appendicitis. Given his nonverbal clues, he appears to be in a great deal of pain. He is accompanied by his father, who does not appear to understand English although José does.

1. You need to ask questions to begin the history and physical exam. Do you ask José the questions or the accompanying parent? Why?
2. How do you begin to build rapport with a school-aged child?
3. José needs to go to surgery quickly. How will you explain this process to him? To his father?
4. The parent seem to be very frightened and, in turn, is scaring José. What is the best approach to address this situation?

Exercise 3

Madison is a 15-year-old girl who presents to the clinic for her annual well-child checkup. She is accompanied by her mother. Madison has several piercings and three visible tattoos (two on her arm and one on her foot). The mother starts complaining about her daughter being "wild" as they are walking down the hall to the exam room.

1. Do you conduct the visit with the mother in the room or ask her to leave?
2. How do you start this history and physical exam?
3. Building rapport with a teenager can be difficult. What are some communication techniques you would use?
4. Madison would like to have the human papillomavirus (HPV) vaccine and obtain birth control. Do you need the mother's consent? What education would you provide along with these medications?
5. The visit is concluding and the mother takes you aside to ask what went on during the visit. How much do you tell her based on the confidentiality guidelines?

Exercise 4

Connor is an 11-year-old boy who has just been admitted to the hospital to start chemotherapy for his newly diagnosed acute lymphoblastic leukemia. The parents do not want Connor to know he has leukemia. They have told him he has a "blood infection" and do not want you to say the words "cancer," "leukemia," or "chemotherapy" in front of him. They conduct all meetings with the providers outside of his room in the hall. You need to do a spinal tap to obtain some cerebrospinal fluid and administer intrathecal methotrexate.

1. How do you explain this to Connor? How do you begin this procedure?
2. Connor is in the gifted program at school. Do you think he believes his parents' explanation that he has a blood infection?
3. What is the problem with not telling Connor the truth?
4. When his parents are out of the room, Connor asks you if he has cancer. What do you tell him?

REVIEW QUESTIONS

1. With regard to exercise 4, Connor's parents keep calling his leukemia an "infection." This is an example of:

   a. Avoidance language
   b. Ignoring
   c. Distancing language
   d. Pretend listening

2. You are beginning a visit with a 15-year-old boy. He is sitting with his arms crossed, looking at the floor. This is an example of:

   a. Attentive listening
   b. Building rapport
   c. Nonverbal communication
   d. Avoidance language

3. You have provided education to your 17-year-old patient regarding the birth control pills you prescribed for her. She has admitted to smoking socially. You discussed the importance of taking the pill at the same time each day as well as not smoking. When you ask her to repeat back what she was taught she talks only about taking the pill at the same time each day and does not mention smoking. This is an example of:

   a. Being nonjudgmental
   b. Selective listening
   c. Distancing language
   d. Paralanguage

4. To convey the impression of attentive listening you should do which of the following:

   a. Sit at the computer, typing in the answers the patient provides into the computer
   b. Stand 3 to 4 feet away from the patient when asking questions
   c. Sit facing the patient, using direct eye contact
   d. Stand over the patient, looking directly at him or her

5. An example of an open-ended question is:

   a. Tell me about the school you go to.
   b. Where is the pain?
   c. Have you vomited today?
   d. Did you have a fever this morning?

6. Which of the following is important when trying to convey empathy?

   a. Sharing your own thoughts and feelings
   b. Providing experiences you have had
   c. Interjecting phrases such as "I understand"
   d. Sympathizing with the patient

7. You are on the phone with a mother about her infant's temperature. Her voice is high pitched and fast, conveying the impression of anxiousness. These vocal elements are an example of:

   a. Paralanguage
   b. Parentese
   c. Distancing language
   d. Nonverbal communication

8. You are taking care of a patient who speaks English but whose parents speak only Spanish. What is your best course of action?

   a. Have the uncle who speaks English interpret the information to the parents
   b. Ask the unit secretary to interpret the information for you
   c. Call a certified interpreter
   d. Allow the patient to translate as the information is not that important

9. When interviewing a teenager, you say "you don't do drugs, right?" This is an example of:

   a. Asking questions to imply blame
   b. An inappropriate use of authority
   c. Providing false assurance
   d. Asking leading questions

10. When examining a toddler it is best to:

    a. Allow the toddler to remain on the parent's lap
    b. Keep all equipment away from the toddler
    c. Have the parent step outside
    d. Talk only to the parent

REFERENCES

Eisenberg, A. M. (2012). *Prescriptive communication for the healthcare provider.* Trafford Publishing.

Hockenberry, M. J. (2011). Communication and physical assessment of the child. In M. J. Hockenberry & D. Wilson (Eds.), *Wong's nursing care of infants and children.* (9th ed., pp. 117–178). St. Louis, MO: Mosby.

Rider, E. A. (2011). Advanced communication strategies for relationship-centered care. *Pediatric Annals, 40* (9), 447–453.

Stein. M. T. (2006). Developmentally based office: Setting the stage for enhanced practice. In S. D. Dixon & M. T. Stein (Eds.), *Encounters with children: Pediatric behavior and development* (4th ed., pp. 72–97). St. Louis, MO: Mosby.

Assessment of the Family

CHAPTER OVERVIEW

The pediatric health care provider must always assess a child within the context of his or her family. This chapter helps the provider to gain greater understanding in examining the family's strengths and weaknesses, in gathering information about the family's medical history, assessing family functioning and relationships, determining the parental knowledge base, and gaining understanding of the family's concerns and needs.

Expected Learning Outcomes

After reading Chiocca, *Advanced Pediatric Assessment, Second Edition,* Chapter 4, the learner will be able to:

1. Assess the child within the context of his or her family
2. Construct a genogram for a child and family
3. Complete a family assessment

Essential Terminology

Adoptive family—a family formed through adoption; can occur in various ways, for example, when a family is created through the adoption of a child, when adopted children join their parents' biologic children, or when stepparents adopt a spouse's children

Family assessment—an element of holistic assessment of child health; helps the provider learn about children through the relationships they have with the people they live with, examine the family's strengths and weaknesses, gather information about the family's medical history, assess family functioning and relationships, determine the parental knowledge base, and gain an understanding of the family's concerns and needs

Foster family—a family in which a child, who is a minor, is placed for either temporary or long-term care; the circumstances leading to the placement vary

Gay- or lesbian-led family—a family in which the head of the household and child's primary caregiver(s) are gay or lesbian, whether married or unmarried

Genogram—a schematic diagram of the family constellation depicting family relationships and medical histories

Grandparent-led family—a family in which the head of the household and child's primary caregiver is the child's grandparent

Single-parent family—a family in which the head of the household and child's primary caregiver is unmarried

Stepfamily—a family in which one parent has children who are not genetically related to the other parent

Two-parent family—a family led by two parents, who may be straight or gay

CRITICAL THINKING EXERCISES

Short-Answer Critical Thinking Exercises

1. What is meant by the term *family demographics*?
2. What is meant by the term *family structure* in the context of a family assessment?
3. Give examples of some different types of family structures.
4. Name some characteristics of healthy families.
5. Discuss some examples of healthy interaction between family members.
6. Explain why assessment of the family is an important component of child health assessment.
7. Name the stages of family development in Wright's Calgary Family Assessment Model.
8. What are some examples of sensitive issues that may arise during a family assessment? What are some ways of dealing with these issues?

Critical Thinking Case Study Exercises

Exercise 1

John, aged 54 years, is married to Maria, aged 53 years. They married in 1998. They have one child, Olivia, aged 14 years, who is in the eighth grade. Olivia was adopted from Guatemala. John's mother, Agnes, is 80 and has diabetes; his father, Nunzio, is 84 and has diabetes type 2 and hypertension. Maria's father is deceased; he died in 1987 of hypernephroma. Her mother has rheumatoid arthritis, hypothyroidism, and chronic fatigue syndrome. John has an older sister (aged 58) who has chronic fatigue syndrome. Maria has five younger siblings; three sisters and two brothers. One sister and one brother have asthma; two sisters have hypothyroidism.

1. Construct a genogram for the Signorelli family.

Exercise 2

Choose a family that you know and conduct a family assessment using the Calgary Family Assessment Model.

Exercise 3

During her annual health supervision visit, 15-year-old Emma Flynn states that she feels like running away from home. When asked why, she says that her mother recently got married after dating a man for only 6 months, and after being single for 10 years. Emma sees her biologic father every other weekend, but he is remarried with three young children. His job requires frequent international travel, and it is difficult for Emma to reach him via phone because of time zone differences. Emma states that she feels that she is at the bottom of everyone's priority list.

1. What type of family assessment should be conducted on Emma's family?
2. Should the assessment be conducted on just Emma, her mother, and her new stepfather, or should her noncustodial, biologic father and his spouse and children be included?
3. What would some priority assessments be?
4. How does Emma's family seem to function?
5. What are the family's teaching needs?

REVIEW QUESTIONS

1. Which of the following statements is true about family assessment?

    a. Questions about parental marital status are considered personal and off-limits
    b. Only certain types of families can be assessed, due to their structure
    c. It is a process, not just the completion of an assessment tool
    d. Changes in the family composition are irrelevant once the initial assessment has been completed

2. Clarity and continuity of communication in healthy families is demonstrated as:

    a. Displaying a no-tolerance policy for any sibling rivalry
    b. Discouraging displays of frustration
    c. Having a family leader who manages all problem solving
    d. Parents who regularly communicate about their philosophy of child-rearing and parenting style

3. The structural assessment of a family includes assessment of:

    a. Who comprises the family and the connection among members
    b. How individuals behave in relation to one another in everyday living
    c. Each family member's medical history
    d. Family religion and ethnicity

4. What is an example of a question regarding internal structure of the family?

    a. Has anyone recently moved in or out? If so, how has this move affected the family?
    b. Do both parents of the family live at home? If not, where do they live?
    c. How often do the children have contact with the parent or parents who do not live at home?
    d. How often is there contact with the extended family (e.g., aunts, uncles)

5. A family in which a minor is placed for either temporary or long-term care is termed a(n):

   a. Adoptive family
   b. Foster family
   c. Blended family
   d. Step-family

6. A schematic diagram of the family showing family relationships and their medical histories is a:

   a. Structural family assessment
   b. Genogram
   c. Genealogy
   d. Internal family assessment

7. What is an example of a question regarding external structure of the family?

   a. If someone in the family was troubled, ill, or depressed, to whom would they be likely to speak?
   b. Which family members live at home?
   c. Are there step-relatives in the family?
   d. How are problems solved in the family?

8. Healthy families are more likely than unhealthy families to:

   a. Negotiate topics for discussion
   b. Have one designated decision maker
   c. Use corporal punishment
   d. Have variable mealtimes

9. In healthy families, adult and child roles, responsibilities, and boundaries are clearly defined. Which of the following examples illustrates this?

   a. Parents do not restrict television, allowing the children to make their own decisions
   b. The children have computers in their rooms so that they can browse the Internet without their parents
   c. Older children consistently care for the younger children while the parents work long hours
   d. Television time for children is limited

10. Of the following, choose the circumstance in which a *comprehensive* family assessment would be indicated.

    a. The family just moved due to a change in a parent's job
    b. The child's teacher calls child protective services because of suspicious bruises
    c. The mother just gave birth to her second child
    d. The father's mother is visiting from her home country

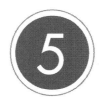

Cultural Assessment of Children and Families

CHAPTER OVERVIEW

This chapter discusses the characteristics of culture, cultural relativism, and cultural competence. In order to provide quality health care to children and their families, the health care provider must be aware of diverse cultural beliefs about health and illness, and be sensitive to the values, beliefs, and health practices among other cultures. This chapter also discusses how the health care provider can deliver culturally competent health care by providing effective communication, overcoming language barriers, avoiding biases and stereotypes, and obtaining a thorough cultural assessment.

Expected Learning Outcomes

After reading Chiocca, *Advanced Pediatric Assessment, Second Edition*, Chapter 5, the learner will be able to:

1. Discuss the basic characteristics of culture
2. Compare and contrast race, ethnicity, and culture
3. Define and discuss cultural relativism
4. Explicate cultural competence in the health care setting
5. Discuss how time orientation differs from culture to culture
6. Compare and contrast various cultural differences regarding nonverbal communication
7. Explain cultural differences in verbal language expression
8. Discuss the importance of the medical interpreter in the health care setting and explain when use of the interpreter is necessary
9. Compare and contrast various cultural differences involving family relationships and child-rearing practices
10. Discuss the importance of modesty in various cultures
11. Identify and explain the three major belief systems regarding the causes of illness
12. Compare and contrast various folk illnesses, traditional health practices, and traditional healers, including the cultural groups they represent
13. Define and discuss culture shock
14. Perform a history and physical examination on immigrant and refugee children
15. Perform a cultural assessment on a child and family

Essential Terminology

Acculturation—the process of adapting to a new culture, while changing many aspects of one's own culture

Alternative medicine—also known as *complementary* or *folk medicine*; includes treatments such as herbs, acupuncture, energy healing, spiritual therapies, or meditation

Assimilation—the process of incorporating the traits of a new culture into one's own culture

Bicultural—facility in two or more cultures, including norms, language, and so forth

Complementary medicine—also known as *alternative* or *folk medicine*; includes treatments such as herbs, acupuncture, energy healing, spiritual therapies, or meditation

Cultural bias—a preference for one's own cultural values and beliefs

Cultural competence—the ability to effectively understand, interact, and communicate with people across all cultures; requires an awareness of one's own culture and worldview, as well as those of other cultures and worldviews

Culture—the learned, shared, and transmitted values, beliefs, norms, and lifeways of a particular group (Leininger, 2001)

Culture-bound syndrome—an illness that is culturally defined; it does not have signs or symptoms that are universally recognizable from a biomedical or scientific perspective and may not be perceived as an illness by another cultural group; also known as a *folk illness*

Culture shock—the disorientation and confusion resulting from leaving one's homeland and coming to a new country with an unfamiliar culture, language, mores, and lifeways

Ethnicity—a group based on common ancestry, history, traditions, language, national origin and, in some cases, common race, and religion

Ethnocentrism—the belief of superiority is one's own race, ethnic group, religion, or sexual orientation

Folk healer—a nonmedical individual who practices healing using traditional methods of healing, for example, herbs, spiritual or religious rituals, laying on of hands, and so forth

Folk illness—an illness that is culturally defined; it does not have signs or symptoms that are universally recognizable from a biomedical or scientific perspective and may not be perceived as an illness by another cultural group; also known as a *culture-bound syndrome*

Folk medicine—also known as *alternative* or *complementary medicine*; includes treatments such as herbs, acupuncture, energy healing, spiritual therapies, or meditation; usually performed by a folk healer

Immigrant—an individual who moves from one country to another, seeking permanent residence in the new country

Lifeways—the way of life, customs, and manner of living of a cultural group

Minority group—a sociological group (e.g., ethnic, racial, religious, gender, sexual orientation) that numbers less than those in the social majority; those in the social majority hold more power in a society than those in the minority group

Mores—the accepted social conventions, customs, and values of a particular cultural group

Multiculturalism—an ideology that advocates that society consist of many different racial, ethnic, and religious groups, and that these groups coexist together in harmony, both integrating into the larger society while keeping the identities of their heritage

Norms—learned behaviors within a cultural group that are determined by the cultural values held by that group

Prejudice—preconceived, often negative notions or stereotypes about all persons belonging to a particular group (e.g., race, gender, ethnicity, sexual orientation)

Race—the biologic classification of people who share the same genetically inherited features such as hair, skin, and eye color

Racism—the belief that one race is superior or inferior to another

Refugee—an individual who has fled from his or her home country and cannot return because of a genuine fear of persecution based on religion, race, nationality, political opinion, or membership in a particular social group (U.S. Department of Homeland Security, 2013)

Stereotype—the assumption that all people belonging to a particular group share all the same characteristics (e.g., values, beliefs, political opinions, etc.)

Subculture—a smaller cultural group within a larger cultural group

Taboo—a strong cultural prohibition against words, actions, or behavior that is considered offensive or forbidden to the cultural group

Traditional healing practice—various methods of prevention, diagnosis, and treatment of illnesses used by folk healers; may include herbs, spiritual or religious rituals, exercises, or other manual therapies

Values—beliefs, attitudes, and behaviors that guide one's actions

Worldview—the perspective from which an individual views the world

CRITICAL THINKING EXERCISES

Short-Answer Critical Thinking Exercises

1. Discuss why there is no universal definition of culture.
2. What is cultural relativism and how does this apply to health care? Give examples.
3. Why and how do poverty and socioeconomic status influence child health? Discuss poverty as a culture.
4. Why does the traditional healing practice of herbal therapy pose a safety concern when used to treat infants or children?

5. Discuss the process by which culture can affect a child's physical and psychosocial health and development.
6. What are some religious and spiritual practices related to birth, death, health, and healing?
7. Define culture shock and give examples of signs that someone may be suffering from it.
8. When providing care to children and families with limited English language abilities, why is it essential for the health care provider to secure a trained interpreter? Why is it undesirable to utilize a child for translation during health care visits?
9. Define and discuss cultural competence.
10. Discuss why the health care provider must be aware of cultural differences regarding nonverbal communication.
11. Compare and contrast the stressors related to culture shock versus those experienced by political refugees. How are these stressors worse when experienced by a child?

Critical Thinking Case Study Exercises

Exercise 1

Sebastian is a 4-year-old boy whose family has recently moved to the United States from Jamaica. Sebastian's mother brought him to the clinic, reporting a 3-day history of fever, cough, and sore throat. When the health care provider lifts Sebastian's shirt to auscultate his posterior chest, she sees bruises in various stages of healing. Based on this, the provider then inspects Sebastian's entire body and finds more bruises in various stages of healing on his sacral region and buttocks. When the provider asks Sebastian's mother how he was hurt, she calmly and readily states that she and Sebastian's father use a belt or shoe to hit him when he misbehaves. When the provider tells the mother that this is considered physical abuse and therefore reportable to Child Protective Services, she appears surprised and astonished.

1. What is cultural relativism and how does it apply in this scenario?
2. Discuss cultural relativism and ethnocentrism.
3. What are some examples of ethnocentrism in pediatric health care?
4. Are there instances in which a child's rights supersede cultural relativism?
5. Are Sebastian's injuries reportable to child protective services or are they within the realm of what is culturally acceptable? Why or why not?

Exercise 2

Juliette is a 2-year-old girl whose mother brings her to the clinic accompanied by her 10-year-old sister. Juliette and her family arrived in the United States from Congo 4 weeks ago and speak only French and Lungala. Juliette needs a physical exam in order to attend day care.

1. In what language should the visit be conducted? If the health care provider does not speak either language, what should be done?
2. What specific parts of the physical examination must the provider be certain to include?

3. In addition to the customary history and physical examination, what other assessments should be made?
4. Is there anything in Juliette's social history that is relevant?

Exercise 3

Three-year-old Juan and his family have recently emigrated from Mexico. His parents brought him to the clinic for a well-child examination. Juan's past medical history reveals that he had one emergency room (ER) visit 2 months ago for vomiting, diarrhea, and abdominal pain. Juan's parents first brought him to a *curandero* (folk healer) who treated him with *azarcon*, and when his condition did not improve, brought him to the ER where he received an intravenous saline bolus. Juan's parents say that when they lived in Mexico, Juan had frequent episodes of diarrhea for which he received azarcon.

1. Given the history of azarcon use more than once with Juan, what specific assessments should be made?
2. What specific condition(s) is/are a concern?
3. Based on the information in the case, what laboratory test(s), if any, should be obtained on Juan?
4. Should Juan's parents be discouraged from using folk healers? Why or why not?
5. Why is it important for the health care provider to become familiar with and be non-judgmental about traditional healing practices?

Exercise 4

Amran, aged 17, is a refugee from Somalia who arrived in the United States 2 weeks ago. She is a Sunni Muslim and speaks both Arabic and Somali, but no English. Amran comes to the student health clinic accompanied by another female student who is acting as an interpreter. Amran is crying and holding her abdomen. Her classmate states that Amran is currently experiencing severe dysmenorrhea, menorrhagia, and some dysuria with prolonged urination. All vital signs are within normal limits. On physical examination, Amran has mild to moderate suprapubic tenderness with no guarding or rebound. No masses are palpable. Inspection of Amran's external genitalia reveals significant keloid formation and a midline fusion of the labia minora, indicating infibulation, thus prohibiting a speculum or bimanual examination.

1. What other historical data should be obtained from Amran?
2. What part of Amran's social history is it important to know?
3. How should the rest of the genitourinary/gynecologic examination proceed? What should be assessed?
4. What, if any, laboratory tests should be obtained?
5. Why is it essential for health care providers to have an awareness and understanding of female genital cutting?
6. How does cultural relativism apply in this scenario? Does the cultural significance of the practice of female genital cutting outweigh Amran's rights? Why or why not?
7. Should Amran be provided with any follow-up care?

REVIEW QUESTIONS

1. Characteristics of culture include all of the following *except:*

    a. Social norms, values, and beliefs
    b. Learned, transmitted by family, peers, and society
    c. Stability over time
    d. Integrated throughout all aspects of a person's life

2. A cultural assessment of the child and family involves:

    a. The process of assisting patients having different cultural orientations
    b. An assessment of a patient's dominant culture, including the accompanying health beliefs, and beliefs about birth, illness, and death
    c. An assessment of potential biologic variations that occur in people of a particular race
    d. Assessment of whether the child and family have sought care from a traditional healer, and advise them to avoid such healers

3. Cultural competence in the health care setting includes which of the following on the part of the health care provider?

    a. Adopting or incorporating traits from other cultures into one's own culture
    b. Changing one's own cultural beliefs to adapt to those of the patients
    c. Providing health care to immigrant and refugee populations
    d. Having an awareness of the role that one's culture plays in health and health care

4. An individual who leaves his or her country of birth due to fear of prosecution based on race, religion, nationality, or politics is a(n):

    a. Immigrant
    b. Refugee
    c. Minority
    d. Cultural broker

5. A mother and her three children have recently arrived in the United States from Congo. The mother reports that her middle child, 10-year-old Helene, has been experiencing bouts of crying, inability to concentrate at school, sleeplessness, and poor appetite. All of the following should be included in the differential diagnoses *except:*

    a. Posttraumatic stress disorder
    b. Culture shock
    c. Cultural bias
    d. Bullying

6. Etienne is a 10-year-old who has recently arrived in the United States from a developing country. When conducting the initial assessment of his history and physical exam, the health care provider should focus on all of the following *except:*

    a. Assessing for signs and symptoms of infectious disease
    b. A nutrition and dental assessment

    c. Signs and symptoms of posttraumatic stress disorder

    d. English language milestones

7. An 8-month-old infant is brought to the clinic by her mother with a 3-day history of cough, fever, runny nose, and difficulty sleeping at night. The family is from Mexico and the infant's mother speaks very little English. In order to assess and treat this child, the provider's *best* action would be to:

    a. Ask an older sibling who is in the clinic room to translate

    b. Secure a trained, bilingual Spanish-speaking interpreter to assist during the encounter

    c. Try to complete as much of the visit as possible in English

    d. Refer the child to a clinic with Spanish-speaking health care providers

8. In which cultural group is the head considered sacred; thus, the health care provider should avoid touching the child's head if possible?

    a. Vietnamese

    b. Chinese

    c. Mexican

    d. Guatemalan

9. The health care provider should avoid maintaining direct eye contact in which of the following cultural groups?

    a. African Americans

    b. European Americans

    c. Mexican immigrants

    d. Korean immigrants

10. In which of the following cultural groups is child discipline done verbally and corporal punishment is rare?

    a. African American

    b. Puerto Rican

    c. Cambodian/Laotian

    d. Mexican/Mexican American

11. Which of the following enhances cultural competence?

    a. Investigating the family hierarchy of a specific culture and addressing family members accordingly

    b. Asking "yes" and "no" questions when obtaining the heath history

    c. Avoiding any visual aids as they may confuse the patient if not culturally relevant

    d. Discouraging the use of complementary medicine and folk healers

12. A 2-week-old Mexican neonate is in the clinic for a health maintenance visit. The infant has a red thread bracelet on her left wrist to protect her from the evil eye (*mal de ojo*). The provider is concerned about the possibility of this amulet becoming a choking hazard, but realizes its

cultural importance. Which of the following is the most culturally sensitive approach to minimizing any choking hazard?

a. Instruct the mother to remove the bracelet altogether
b. Instruct the mother to place the bracelet on the infant's non-dominant wrist
c. Instruct the mother to place the bracelet on the infant's ankle
d. Instruct the mother to keep the bracelet in the infant's baby bag

13. Which of the following cultural groups views an overweight infant or child as healthy?

a. European American
b. Mexican/Mexican American
c. Cambodian/Laotian
d. Arab/Arab American

14. When working with children and families from diverse backgrounds, it is essential for the health care provider to know whether any traditional healing practices are used for all of the following reasons *except:*

a. The use of traditional healing practices is reportable to child protective services
b. The use of some traditional healing practices may be potentially harmful to children
c. Traditional healing practices may leave marks and be confused with physical abuse
d. Some traditional healers may reject the use of medications or other biomedical therapies

15. Because of cultural or religious beliefs regarding modesty, adolescent girls having which of the following ethnicities or religions would need to be examined only by a *female* health care provider for a pelvic or external genital examination?

a. African American
b. European American
c. Muslim girl who practices *hijab*
d. Irish American Catholic

16. The holistic perspective on health holds that health and illness are determined by:

a. A disruption in the balance of nature
b. Supernatural forces such as a god or gods, voodoo, witchcraft, or fate
c. Emotions or spirits
d. Viruses, bacteria, or bodily trauma

17. Which of the following folk illnesses involves a traditional method of healing that may be fatal?

a. *Mal de ojo*
b. *Empacho*

    c. *Caida de la mallera*
    d. *Susto*

18. Mothers or grandmothers have the primary role in discipline and child care in all of the following cultures *except:*

    a. African American
    b. Arab/Arab American
    c. Navajo
    d. Puerto Rican

19. Complications of female genital cutting may include:

    a. Infection with herpes virus
    b. Precipitous labor and delivery
    c. Urinary incontinence
    d. Prolonged menstruation

20. Aromatherapy, a form of complementary/alternative medicine, should not be used on a child with which of the following diagnoses?

    a. Asthma
    b. Fractures
    c. Back pain
    d. Anxiety

SAMPLE CULTURAL ASSESSMENT OF THE CHILD AND FAMILY

Patient Name _____ Date of Birth _____ Date _____
Gender _____ Race _____

Cultural group affiliation (e.g., Hmong, Chinese, Mexican)_____

Country of child's birth_____

Arrival to new country (date)_____

Number of adults living in home_____

Relationship of each adult to child

    1. _____   Relationship_____
    2. _____   Relationship_____
    3. _____   Relationship_____
    4. _____   Relationship_____

Number of children living in home and age of each child

    1. _____
    2. _____
    3. _____
    4. _____

Relationship of each child to patient

1. _____   Relationship_____
2. _____   Relationship_____
3. _____   Relationship_____
4. _____   Relationship_____

Language(s) spoken at home

1. _____
2. _____
3. _____

Preferred language for daily communication_____

Can the child/family read in their primary language?

If immigrant, circumstances of immigration_____

Is child/family refugee? _____ Reason for refugee status_____

What type (if any) of community support does the child and family receive?
_____

Is there a particular family member who makes major decisions?
_____

What is the family's religion and how observant are they?
_____

Does the family use a traditional healer?_____

Does the family use any methods of traditional healing themselves (e.g., herbs, amulets, healing rituals)?_____

Does the child/adolescent or family have any concerns about discrimination or racism?_____

REFERENCES

Leininger, M. (Ed.). (2001). *Culture care diversity and universality: A theory of nursing.* Sudbury, MA: Jones and Bartlett.

U. S. Department of Homeland Security. (2013). Refugees. Retrieved September 28, 2014 from http://www.uscis.gov/humanitarian/refugees-asylum/refugees

Obtaining the Pediatric Health History

CHAPTER OVERVIEW

Obtaining an accurate health history is the essential first step in the pediatric health care visit. The accuracy of the physical examination and diagnoses depends on whether the health history is accurate and complete. This chapter helps the student refine skills in obtaining the pediatric health history.

Expected Learning Outcomes

After reading Chiocca, *Advanced Pediatric Assessment, Second Edition*, Chapter 6, the learner will be able to:

1. Identify the type of history that needs to be obtained based on the reason for seeking care
2. Identify how the various components of the health history differ according to age and developmental stage
3. State the optimal setting in which to obtain the health history
4. Demonstrate age and developmentally appropriate communication and interview skills when obtaining the health history
5. Obtain an accurate and complete health history for a pediatric patient
6. Demonstrate the ability to clearly, objectively, and accurately document all historical assessment findings

Essential Terminology

Emergency health history—similar to the focused history; involves the quick collection of data in an acute situation; often done rapidly, usually with simultaneous interventions.

Focused (episodic) health history—a problem-centered history, focusing on the present illness or complaint

Follow-up health history—the history obtained when the child returns to the office after an illness or injury to assess whether the problem is the same, better, or worse

Initial (comprehensive) health history—an initial, comprehensive health history, which creates a database of information for the child who is new to the provider's practice

Interval (well-child) health history—a history that updates the child's health status since the last office visit

CRITICAL THINKING EXERCISES

Short-Answer Critical Thinking Exercises

1. Define and explain the following types of pediatric health histories. Include the indication for each:

   a. Initial (comprehensive) health history
   b. Interval (well-child) health history
   c. Focused (episodic) health history
   d. Follow-up health history
   e. Emergency health history

2. Explain how each type of health history is not necessarily mutually exclusive.
3. Which components of the health history are common to all types of pediatric health histories?
4. What are the components of the prenatal, birth and neonatal histories? In new patients, these histories should be collected until what age?
5. What is the review of systems (ROS)? In what context should it be done?
6. What is the social history? Why is it particularly important to obtain when working with the pediatric population?
7. What is a family history? How does it differ from the social history? How is it relevant to pediatric health care?
8. What is an interval history? Why do the components of the interval history change so frequently for the pediatric patient?
9. In families for whom English is a second language, why must a trained interpreter be used when obtaining the health history, versus asking the child to interpret?
10. Describe how the pediatric health care provider can assess pain in infants and young children.

Critical Thinking Case Study Exercises

Exercise 1: Initial Health History

Mariana is a 3-year-old girl who is new to the clinic, having recently moved to the area from Mexico with her parents. She is accompanied by both her parents and her 1-year-old brother. Mariana is at the clinic for a full physical exam. Her parents speak only Spanish. Fill in these blanks with the questions you would ask during the visit. Add any questions that are not included but are important to include.

Subjective Data

Biographical data: _____

Source of information: _____

Reason for seeking care: _____

Past medical history (PMH):
  Prenatal history: _____

  Birth history: _____

  Neonatal history: _____

Past illnesses: _____

Past hospitalizations (dates, reason[s]): _____
  Injuries/Ingestions (intentional/unintentional injuries; dates of injuries/ ingestions): _____
  Emergency department visits (note date, age of child, and reason for visit):

_____

Past surgeries (dates, type of surgery): _____

Current medications: _____

Immunizations: _____

Screening procedures done: _____

Family medical history:

Allergies:

Review of Systems

  General: _____
  Integument: _____
  Head: _____
  Eyes: _____
  Nose: _____
  Ears: _____
  Mouth: _____
  Throat: _____
  Neck: _____
  Nodes: _____
  Chest: _____
  Respiratory: _____
  Cardiovascular: _____
  Gastrointestinal: _____
  Genitourinary: _____
  Gynecologic: _____
  Musculoskeletal: _____
  Neurologic: _____
  Endocrine: _____
  Lymphatic: _____

Nutrition: _____

Elimination: _____

Safety: _____

Sleep: _____

Social: _____

Growth and development: _____

Exercise 2: Interval Health History

You asked Mariana's parents to bring her back to the clinic in 2 months for re-assessment. Using the space provided here, and referring to exercise #1, record what historical questions you would ask.

_____

_____

_____

Exercise 3: Focused History

Billy is a 15-month-old toddler brought to the clinic by his mother. She says that Billy has a 2-day history of irritability, runny nose, decreased appetite, and fever. Fill in the blanks to complete the focused history.

Reason for seeking care: _____

History of present illness (HPI): _____

Onset (date, time, sudden versus gradual): _____

Duration: _____

Characteristics and course of signs and symptoms: _____

Activating/aggravating/precipitating factors: _____

Relieving factors: _____

Allergies: _____

Current medications (include over-the-counter [OTC] and prescription meds, and alternative therapies taken; include exact dose, frequency, and time of last dose given): _____

Immunization status: _____

Recent illnesses, sick contacts: _____

ROS/chronic illnesses: _____

Exercise 4: Follow-Up

You ask Billy's mother to bring him back for a re-check in 2 days. Use the space provided here to complete the follow-up history.

_____

_____

_____

Exercise 5: Emergency History

A 6-year-old child presents to the emergency department with his mother. The school nurse had called, reporting that the child fell off the jungle gym during school recess. Use the space provided here to indicate what questions should be obtained for the emergency history.

_____

_____

_____

REVIEW QUESTIONS

1. Children are usually brought for health care by a parent. At what age would it be appropriate to begin to question the child about presenting symptoms?

   a. 2 years
   b. 3 years
   c. 5 years
   d. 7 years

2. The nurse practitioner reading a medical record sees the following notation: "One emergency department visit for laceration to the right arm after falling on broken glass." This is an example of:

   a. Past history
   b. Review of systems
   c. Functional assessment
   d. Reason for seeking care (chief complaint)

3. When taking a health history for a child, what information in addition to that for an adult, is usually obtained?

   a. Allergies and current medications
   b. Developmental milestones achieved
   c. Environmental hazards
   d. Hospitalization history

4. Which of the following histories should be obtained when a child is being seen for the first time?

   a. Interval history
   b. Focused history
   c. Initial history
   d. Follow-up history

5. The past history includes:

   a. Hospitalizations
   b. Social history
   c. Family history
   d. Nutrition history

6. The family history includes:

   a. The health history of the child's parents and siblings
   b. The family's current living conditions
   c. Whether one or both parents work outside the home
   d. Determining who the child's primary caregiver is

7. You are seeing a 10-year-old child who has been your patient since birth. The type of history that would be obtained from this ambulatory, apparently well child during a health maintenance visit would be:

   a. Complete health history
   b. Episodic health history
   c. Interval history
   d. Emergency history

8. The medical assistant documents the following in the electronic medical record: "Mother states that child has a red, round itchy spot on her arm." This is an example of:

   a. Initial health history
   b. Reason for seeking care (also chief complaint)
   c. Review of systems
   d. Past medical history

9. Which of the following is an example of subjective data?

   a. "Wheezes heard throughout all lung fields"
   b. "No retractions noted"
   c. "He has had a cough for a week now and is using his inhaler more."
   d. "Copious, thick, green nasal discharge seen on inspection"

10. Which of the following is an example of objective data?

   a. "Abdomen distended; child lying on right side, guarding abdomen"
   b. "Mother states child woke up this morning with generalized abdominal pain"
   c. "Child now says that pain is in right lower quadrant (RLQ)"
   d. "Child states he is nauseated and feels like vomiting"

11. A child's neonatal history should be obtained for which of the following ages?

   a. Age 3 years and younger
   b. Age 4 years and younger
   c. Age 5 years and younger
   d. Age 6 years and younger

12. A component of the neonatal history is assessment of:

   a. Timing of onset of prenatal care
   b. Assessment of medications taken during pregnancy
   c. Length of labor
   d. Apgar score

13. A family history includes assessment of:

   a. History of diabetes
   b. Whether the family is immigrant or natural-born
   c. Family's socioeconomic status
   d. Which individuals live in the home

14. The acronym, BIHEADSS is used as a guideline to obtain the social history. For which age group is this acronym typically used?

   a. Infant
   b. Toddler/preschooler
   c. School-aged child
   d. Adolescent

15. Depending on the clinical situation, the nurse may establish one of four types of a database. An episodic database is described as:

   a. Including a complete health history and full physical examination
   b. Concerning mainly one problem
   c. Evaluation of a previously identified problem
   d. Rapid collection of data in conjunction with lifesaving measures

Assessing Safety and Injury Risk in Children

CHAPTER OVERVIEW

This chapter helps the learner to become adept in performing an age- and developmentally appropriate injury risk assessment of children from birth through adolescence, to identify potential risks for injury, and to accurately record the assessment findings.

Expected Learning Outcomes

After reading Chiocca, *Advanced Pediatric Assessment, Second Edition*, Chapter 7, the learner will be able to:

1. Explicate the importance of the injury risk assessment in the pediatric population
2. Identify relevant safety assessments according to age and developmental stage
3. Compare and contrast risks for injury according to age and developmental stage
4. Discuss how the characteristics of the child, parent, and environment can interact to increase or decrease risk of injury to a child

Essential Terminology

Active injury prevention strategy—interventions to prevent injury that require action on the part of the parent or child

Haddon's matrix—an epidemiological tool used to assess injury risk and devise strategies for prevention

Morbidity—related to illness

Mortality—related to death

Passive injury prevention strategy—interventions to prevent injury that require no action on the part of the parent or child

Risk factor—a variable associated with an increased likelihood of developing a disease or injury

CRITICAL THINKING EXERCISES

Short-Answer Critical Thinking Exercises

1. Discuss why injury risk assessment is such a crucial part of pediatric health assessment.
2. Define morbidity and mortality. Why do the causes of morbidity and mortality differ among children living in rural versus urban areas?
3. Compare and contrast the causes of morbidity and mortality in children living in developed and developing countries.
4. Discuss what is meant by "the new morbidity." What assessments should be made to determine a child's vulnerability to the new morbidity?
5. What are the developmental risk factors for injury by age group? Why are these risk factors different according to a child's age and developmental stage?
6. What are some risk factors for injury to a child related to parenting style? Explain.
7. What are some environmental risk factors for child injury?
8. What are non-modifiable risk factors for injury to children? Explain why they change according to a child's age and developmental stage.
9. What are the universal pediatric safety assessments?
10. What are the pediatric safety assessments according to age and developmental stage? Why are these assessments different according to a child's age and developmental stage?
11. Pick a common childhood injury and use Haddon's matrix to consider potential risk factors and prevention strategies.
12. Why is it important to ask about a history of previous injuries during the safety assessment?

Critical Thinking Case Study Exercise

Exercise 1

During a well-child examination, when asked, the parents of a 3-year-old child state that they have several firearms in the home.

1. What follow-up questions should be asked about the guns?

Exercise 2

During the health maintenance visit, the mother of an 18-month-old child states that the child is "very busy" and it is hard for her to "keep up" with the child since she has a newborn at home who consumes much of her time. The mother also says that she is very sleep-deprived because she is nursing and the baby wakes every 2 hours to feed.

1. What, if any, risks for injury exist for both children in this scenario?
2. Why would one or both of these children be at high risk for injury?
3. What specific injury risk assessments should be made on the toddler?
4. What specific injury risk assessments should be made on the newborn?

Exercise 3

Annie is a 15-year-old who is in the office for her annual physical. She is accompanied by her mother.

1. Are injury risk assessments still relevant for a 15-year-old?
2. If so, what specific assessments should be made?
3. Is it better to have Annie's mother in or out of the exam room during the injury risk assessment? Why or why not?

Exercise 4

Three children from one family are brought to the clinic for school physicals accompanied by their mother. When asked whether anyone in the home smokes cigarettes, the mother replies that both she and the children's father smoke, but they always smoke outside.

1. What, if any, risks for injury exist for the children in this scenario?
2. What other assessments should be made?
3. What specific parent education should be provided?

REVIEW QUESTIONS

1. The leading cause of death in American children is:

   a. Unintentional injury
   b. Homicide
   c. Suicide
   d. Cancer

2. Violence and injuries are the leading cause of death among children living in the United States. Of all fatal unintentional injuries in the pediatric population, which of the following is the *leading* cause of mortality?

   a. Gun-related injuries
   b. Traumatic brain injuries
   c. Motor vehicle–related injuries
   d. Drowning

3. In order of frequency, the top three causes of death in American children aged 1 to 4 years are:

   a. Unintentional injury, sudden infant death syndrome, congenital anomalies
   b. Congenital anomalies, unintentional injury, sudden infant death syndrome
   c. Sudden infant death syndrome, unintentional injury, homicide
   d. Unintentional injury, congenital anomalies, homicide

4. In infants until age 2 years, head circumference exceeds chest circumference. The clinical implications of this include all of the following *except*:

   a. Increased risk of traumatic brain injury
   b. Increased risk of whiplash injury
   c. Increased risk of drowning
   d. Increased risk of aspiration

5. A risk factor that predisposes a child to unintentional injury is:

   a. Female gender
   b. Authoritarian parenting style
   c. Poverty
   d. High level of parental education

6. A developmental characteristic that increases risk for injury in a 6-month-old infant includes all of the following *except*:

   a. Poor head control
   b. Crying
   c. Putting objects in the mouth
   d. Creeping and crawling

7. A developmental characteristic that increases risk for injury in a 2-year-old includes:

   a. Poor pincer grasp
   b. Temper tantrums
   c. Poor head control
   d. Desire to be less independent

8. Which of the following children is at highest risk of injury?

   a. A 2-week-old infant in a vehicle restraint in the rear seat of the car, facing forward
   b. A 3-year-old playing with toy cars with small wheels
   c. A 13-month-old toddler who sleeps prone
   d. A group of six 14-year-olds in a backyard pool with a parent on the patio

9. An example of a passive strategy to prevent injuries in children is:

   a. The use of a car seat
   b. The use of window guards
   c. The use of childproof caps on medication bottles
   d. The use of electrical outlet covers

10. When conducting a safety assessment of a 4-year-old, which of the following assessments is *most* relevant?

   a. Ask about a childproofed environment
   b. Ask about choking hazards
   c. Ask whether the child and parent co-sleep
   d. Ask whether the child uses a bicycle helmet

11. A 1-year-old child is vulnerable to head injuries because children at this age have:

    a. Poor head control
    b. A large head in proportion to the body
    c. Increased gross motor abilities that include running and climbing
    d. Increased risk-taking behaviors

12. A safety assessment of a school-aged child would include all of the following *except*:

    a. Inquiring about the use of seatbelts
    b. Inquiring about the use of bicycle helmets
    c. Inquiring about whether pot handles are turned toward the rear of the stove
    d. Inquiring about the child's knowledge of "stranger danger"

13. When conducting a safety assessment of an adolescent, the teen should be reassured that whatever he or she discusses with the provider will not be shared with the parent or caregiver unless the teen:

    a. Discloses regular marijuana use
    b. Demonstrates a safety threat to himself or others
    c. Discloses that she is sexually active
    d. Discloses only occasional seatbelt use

14. During the safety assessment portion of a well-child visit, which of the following statements made by the parent of a 10-year-old child is a red flag for the need for parental injury prevention education?

    a. "We never let her swim in a lake or ocean."
    b. "She didn't begin swimming lessons until she was 6 years old."
    c. "We don't let our kids dive into our backyard pool."
    d. "She is an excellent swimmer, so we let her and her friends swim in our backyard pool by themselves."

15. Universal safety assessment in the pediatric patient includes all of the following *except*:

    a. Assessment of choking hazards
    b. Assessment of secondhand smoke exposure
    c. Assessment of safe storage of firearms in the home
    d. Assessment of motor vehicle safety

16. According to the American Academy of Pediatrics guidelines (2011), it is recommended that a child remain seated in a lap-and-shoulder booster seat in a vehicle until the child is:

    a. 4 feet, 5 inches in height or between ages 8 and 10 years
    b. 4 feet, 9 inches in height or between ages 8 and 12 years
    c. 80 pounds in weight or between ages 8 and 12 years
    d. 50 pounds in weight or between ages 4 and 5 years

17. The American Academy of Pediatrics states that which of the following should not be provided to children under any circumstances?

    a. Skateboards
    b. Trampolines
    c. Scooters
    d. Roller blades

18. During a routine health care visit, the parent of a 5-year-old asks about street safety, stating that the child is very independent and does not like to hold hands when crossing the street. The parent wants to know if it is safe to let the child cross the street independently. The provider responds that when crossing the street, an adult should hold a child's hand until:

    a. 5 years of age
    b. 6 years of age
    c. 7 years of age
    d. 8 years of age

19. Which of the following statements regarding gun safety is *untrue*:

    a. All firearms should be stored in a locked container
    b. All firearms in the home should be unloaded
    c. Children who live in rural areas have been taught how to handle firearms and are at very low risk for gun-related injury
    d. BB, pellet, and paint-ball guns can cause serious injuries to children

20. According to the American Academy of Pediatrics guidelines (2011), which of the following statements regarding automobile safety for children is correct?

    a. Children younger than age 2 years may ride in a car seat facing either the front or the rear of the car, depending on weight
    b. Children who weigh 40 pounds or more (18.2 kg) may use adult-type restraints
    c. A child may ride in the front seat once he or she has reached 12 years of age
    d. Infants younger than age 2 years should ride in restraint devices facing the rear of the vehicle

SAMPLE DOCUMENTATION: SAFETY ASSESSMENT

The Safety and Risk Reduction Assessment is age specific. Use the following table as an assessment tool by finding the child's age in the left-hand column, then making the corresponding safety assessments in the right-hand column. Make a check mark beside each completed assessment, and include any notations regarding more in-depth assessments that may be required, as well as necessary child and parent education.

AGE	INJURY RISK ASSESSMENTS
0–6 months	• Burns • Falls • Sleep position • Crib safety • Shaking • Stings around neck • Car safety seat • Sun exposure • Carbon monoxide/smoke detectors • Smoke-free environment • Home safety/emergency plan
6–12 months	• Burns • Falls • Choking • Kitchen safety • Crib safety • Poisoning prevention • Lead poisoning • Walkers • Choking hazards • Shaking • Stings around neck • Appropriate child supervision • Water safety/drowning prevention • Car seat safety • Gun safety • Sun exposure • Carbon monoxide/smoke detectors • Smoke-free environment • Home safety/emergency plan
1–2 years	• Burns • Falls • Choking • Poisoning prevention • Kitchen safety • Sharp objects • Shaking • Stings around neck • Crib safety • Lead poisoning • Walkers • Appropriate child supervision • Safe play area • Water safety/drowning prevention

(continued)

AGE	INJURY RISK ASSESSMENTS
	• Car seat safety • Gun safety • Sun exposure • Carbon monoxide/smoke detectors • Smoke-free environment • Home safety/emergency plan
2 years	• Burns • Falls • Choking • Shaking • Stings around neck • Poisoning prevention • Kitchen safety • Window safety • Lead poisoning • Appropriate child supervision • Safe play area • Pedestrian safety • Water safety/drowning prevention • Car seat safety • Gun safety • Animal safety • Sun exposure • Carbon monoxide/smoke detectors • Smoke-free environment • Home safety/emergency plan
3–4 years	• Choking • Poisoning prevention • Kitchen safety • Window safety • Lead poisoning • Appropriate child supervision • Safe play area • Pedestrian safety • Water safety/drowning prevention • Car seat safety • Gun safety • Animal safety • Safety helmets/use of protective gear • Sun exposure • Carbon monoxide/smoke detectors • Smoke-free environment • Home safety/emergency plan
5–6 years	• Seatbelts/vehicle restraints • Booster seat • Knowing child's friends

AGE	INJURY RISK ASSESSMENTS
	• Gun safety • Pedestrian safety • Monitor computer/screen time • Safe play area • Pedestrian safety • Water/swimming safety • Sports/play safety • Sun exposure • Safety helmets/use of protective gear • Sexual safety ("good touch/bad touch") • Carbon monoxide/smoke detectors • Smoke-free environment • Home safety/emergency plan
7–8 years	• Seatbelts/vehicle restraints • Booster seat • Knowing child's friends • Gun safety • Pedestrian safety • Safe play area • Monitor computer/screen time • Water/swimming safety • Sun exposure • Sports/play safety • Safety helmets/use of protective gear • Sexual safety ("good touch/bad touch") • Carbon monoxide/smoke detectors • Smoke-free environment • Home safety/emergency plan
9–10 years	• Seatbelts/vehicle restraints • Booster seat • Knowing child's friends • Gun safety • Monitor computer/screen time • Water/swimming safety • Safe play area • Sports/play safety • Safety helmets/use of protective gear • Sexual safety ("good touch/bad touch") • Use of alcohol/tobacco • Safe dating/sexual safety • Sun exposure • Carbon monoxide/smoke detectors • Smoke-free environment • Home safety/emergency plan

(continued)

AGE	INJURY RISK ASSESSMENTS
11–14 years	• Seatbelts/vehicle restraints • Booster seat • Knowing child's friends • Gun safety • Monitor computer/screen time • Water/swimming safety • Sports/play safety • Sun exposure • Safety helmets/use of protective gear • Sexual safety ("good touch/bad touch") • Safe dating/sexual safety • Use of alcohol/tobacco/drugs • Carbon monoxide/smoke detectors • Smoke-free environment • Home safety/emergency plan
15–21 years	• Seatbelts/vehicle restraints • Knowing child's friends • Gun safety • Monitor computer/screen time • Water/swimming safety • Sports/play safety • Sun exposure • Safety helmets/use of protective gear • Sexual safety ("good touch/bad touch") • Safe dating/sexual safety • Use of alcohol/tobacco/drugs • Carbon monoxide/smoke detectors • Smoke-free environment • Home safety/emergency plan

REFERENCE

American Academy of Pediatrics Committee on Injury, Violence, and Poison Prevention. (2011). Policy statement: Child passenger safety. *Pediatrics, 127* (4), 788; reaffirmation policy: (2002). *Pediatrics, 109* (3), 550–553.

The Pediatric Physical Examination

CHAPTER OVERVIEW

This chapter serves as an introduction to pediatric physical examination, specifically the developmental aspects of preparing and examining the child, age parameters for vital sign and anthropometric measurements, and the physical examination techniques of inspection, auscultation, palpation, and percussion. The pediatric general survey is also discussed.

Expected Learning Outcomes

After reading Chiocca, *Advanced Pediatric Assessment, Second Edition*, Chapter 8, the learner will be able to:

1. List the equipment and supplies necessary to conduct a physical examination of the pediatric patient
2. Accurately obtain and record vital signs in children, from birth through adolescence, and recognize deviations from normal
3. Accurately obtain and record anthropometric measurements in children, from birth through adolescence, and recognize deviations from normal
4. Discuss developmental considerations related to measuring vital signs and anthropometric measurements in children, from birth through adolescence
5. Discuss the sequencing of the physical examination in children and why it differs according to age, developmental stage, and reason for health care visit
6. Compare and contrast pediatric variations of the four major physical assessment skills: inspection, palpation, percussion, and auscultation
7. Demonstrate the ability to record all physical assessment findings accurately and completely

Essential Terminology

Anthropometry—body measurements, for example, weight, height, length, head circumference, and body mass index

Auscultation—listening to body sounds produced by the airway, lungs, heart, blood vessels, stomach, and intestines; most auscultation requires the use of a stethoscope, although some body sounds can be heard directly

Dullness—a percussion sound, thud-like in quality, soft to medium in intensity, moderate to high pitched, of medium duration; heard over solid organs such as the liver or stomach

Duration—the length of a percussion note

Flatness—a percussion sound, flat in quality, soft in intensity, high pitched, short in duration; heard over bone and muscle

General survey—a cursory head-to-toe assessment conducted before the full, detailed physical assessment

Hyperresonance—a percussion sound; booming in quality, very loud in intensity, very low pitched, long in duration; heard over the lungs of a very young child or lungs with air trapping

Inspection—purposeful, skilled, systematic observation during physical assessment

Intensity—the loudness or the amplitude of a sound; that is, loud or soft

Palpation—the physical examination technique in which the examiner uses touch to gather assessment findings; can be light or deep, depending on the amount of pressure applied

Percussion—the physical examination technique that involves the use of tapping to assess underlying organs and structures

Pitch—the frequency of a sound. A high-pitched sound corresponds to a high-frequency sound wave (e.g., percussion of a gastric air bubble); a low-pitched sound corresponds to a low-frequency sound wave (e.g., percussion over a normal lung)

Quality—the description of a body sound; for example, musical, crackling

Resonance—a percussion sound, hollow in quality, medium to loud in intensity, low pitched, long in duration; heard over the normal lung

Stadiometer—a device for measuring height; most often consists of a vertical ruler with a sliding horizontal rod or paddle that is adjusted to rest at a right angle at the top of the child's head

Tympany—a percussion sound, drum-like in quality, loud in intensity, high pitched, medium duration; heard over the stomach or gastric bubble

CRITICAL THINKING EXERCISES

Short-Answer Critical Thinking Exercises

1. Discuss ways in which the pediatric health care provider prepares for the physical examination for each pediatric age group, from infancy through adolescence.
2. Discuss the components of the pediatric general survey.
3. When assessing younger children, why it is particularly important to begin the physical assessment as soon as possible?

4. What are some factors that affect a child's body temperature, heart rate, and respiratory rate, and why?
5. Why does the sequence of the pediatric physical examination differ depending on the child's age and, in some instances, presenting complaint?
6. What are the six systematic techniques of inspection discussed in Chapter 8? What is the rationale for using these techniques? What is an example of each of these techniques?

Critical Thinking Case Study Exercises

Exercise 1

Ava, a 10-month-old African American toddler, is brought to the clinic by her mother for her health maintenance visit. The health care provider obtains the health history while Ava is held on her mother's lap. Each time the provider makes eye contact with, smiles at, or leans toward Ava, she cries and buries her face in her mother's chest. Now it is time for the physical exam.

1. Is Ava's behavior normal for her age?
2. How should the provider proceed with the exam? What should the next steps be?
3. Where is the best place to conduct Ava's physical exam?
4. In terms of sequencing the exam, in what order should the provider conduct the physical exam?

Exercise 2

Pearl is a 16-month-old Asian American toddler who presents for an episodic visit. She is accompanied by both parents, who state that Pearl has had a cough and runny nose for approximately 5 days. Pearl's parents state that this morning, she "felt hot," became irritable, and began pulling on her ear. Currently, Pearl is irritable, flushed, and crying on and off. A month ago, Pearl had her 15-month health maintenance visit and her physical and developmental examination was unremarkable at that time.

1. Does Pearl need a full head-to-toe exam at this time?
2. Where is the best place for the provider to conduct the physical examination in order to minimize Pearl's anxiety?
3. Because Pearl is irritable, would it be better to ask her parents to step out of the room during the physical examination?
4. Based on the preceding information, in what order should the physical examination be conducted?

Exercise 3

Nick is a 3-year-old boy of European ancestry. He is brought to the clinic by his mother for his annual health examination. While the provider is gathering the health history, Nick is listening and offering his own answers. His mother chuckles at this, telling the provider that she is not surprised at this behavior;

Nick talks nonstop at home and asks "a million questions." The provider notes that Nick's facial expression appears to indicate that he is somewhat frightened as his body functions are discussed.

1. Is Nick's behavior at home as described by his mother developmentally normal or is it concerning? Why or why not?
2. Is it normal for Nick to appear somewhat frightened as he listens to discussions of his bodily functions? Why or why not?
3. For a child Nick's age, should the provider be cognizant of certain words used during the visit? If so, give examples of what kinds of words or phrases should be avoided.
4. Is there anything specific the provider can do to gain a preschooler's cooperation before or during the physical examination?
5. In what sequence should the physical examination be conducted?

Exercise 4

Julia is an 11-year-old girl of European ancestry who is at the clinic for her school physical. She is accompanied by her grandmother who has been her legal guardian since she was 2 years old.

1. When obtaining the health history, who should the provider direct questions to? Julia, her grandmother, or both?
2. In what sequence should the physical examination be conducted?
3. Julia asks questions during the exam. Should the provider answer her questions or defer to her grandmother?
4. Should Julia be given the option to have her grandmother in or out of the room during the physical exam?
5. What are some developmental considerations that the provider must keep in mind when examining a school-aged child?

Exercise 5

Javier is a 16-year-old Mexican American boy whose mother has brought him to the clinic for his annual health maintenance exam. This is his first time at the clinic, and there are only female health care providers.

1. When obtaining the health history, who should the provider direct questions to? Javier, his mother, or both?
2. Are there parts of the history that should definitely be elicited from Javier specifically? If so, which parts? What is the best way to deal with this?
3. Should Javier's mother be in or out of the exam room during the exam?
4. In what sequence should the physical examination be conducted?
5. What special considerations exist for the physical exam as a result of having an opposite sex provider?
6. What tone should the provider take during the exam when speaking to Javier?
7. What are some developmental considerations that the provider must keep in mind when examining adolescents?
8. Discuss privacy and confidentiality as it relates to adolescent health care.

REVIEW QUESTIONS

1. The first step in the physical examination is *always*:

   a. Inspection
   b. Auscultation
   c. Palpation
   d. Percussion

2. The sequence of a physical examination changes to a head-to-toe approach beginning with which age group?

   a. Toddler
   b. Preschooler
   c. School-aged child
   d. Adolescent

3. A 6-year-old boy presents to the clinic with complaints of tactile fever at home and cold symptoms. The nurse is now measuring his vital signs. What is the best way to measure this child's temperature?

   a. Oral
   b. Rectal
   c. Axillary
   d. Tactile

4. When performing a physical examination on a well toddler, which of the following body parts should be examined last?

   a. Heart and lungs
   b. Abdomen and genitals
   c. Ears and throat
   d. Hips and extremities

5. When the health care provider is ready to begin the physical examination, the 2-month-infant patient is asleep. It is best start the physical examination with:

   a. Assessment of the hips
   b. Auscultation of heart, lungs, abdomen
   c. Examination of the tympanic membrane
   d. Elicitation of the Moro reflex

6. In which of the following age groups does gentle handling of and role-play with the provider's equipment (e.g., stethoscope, otoscope) enhance trust and facilitate the physical examination?

   a. Older infants
   b. Toddlers
   c. School-aged children
   d. Adolescents

7. When conducting a physical examination of an older infant, the provider takes the infant from her mother's lap and places her on the exam table. She begins to cry immediately. The provider places the infant back in the mother's lap and the child stops crying, and the provider completes the physical assessment there. Based on knowledge of psychosocial growth and development, this infant's age is likely:

   a. 4 to 5 months
   b. 5 to 6 months
   c. 6 to 7 months
   d. 7 to 8 months

8. Measurement of blood pressure becomes routine at health maintenance visits beginning at age:

   a. 2 years
   b. 3 years
   c. 4 years
   d. 5 years

9. At the 6-month wellness visit, an infant who weighed 2.9 kg at birth would be expected to weigh approximately:

   a. 4 kg
   b. 6 kg
   c. 7 kg
   d. 8 kg

10. All of the following conditions raise body temperature in a child or teen *except*:

   a. Anesthetic agents
   b. Ovulation
   c. Dehydration
   d. Crying

11. During the second year of life, the average child grows approximately:

   a. 6 cm a year
   b. 7 cm a year
   c. 8 cm a year
   d. 10 cm a year

12. Head circumference should be measured routinely as part of the well-child visit in children aged:

   a. 1 year and younger
   b. 2 years and younger
   c. 3 years and younger
   d. 4 years and younger

13. Head and chest circumferences should be equal at:

   a. 6 months of age
   b. 1 year of age

    c. 2 years of age

    d. 3 years of age

14. In children aged 2 years and younger, recumbent height (i.e., length) is measured rather than standing height because of:

    a. Large head size

    b. Physiologic flat feet

    c. Physiologic lordosis

    d. Physiologic kyphosis

15. Deep palpation is used to assess:

    a. Organ position

    b. Skin temperature

    c. Muscle tone

    d. Superficial tenderness

16. Which of the following physical assessment techniques is often used to assess for costovertebral tenderness?

    a. Palpation

    b. Direct percussion

    c. Indirect percussion

    d. Blunt percussion

17. During percussion of the abdomen, the sound produced is dull. This sound is produced by:

    a. Gastric air

    b. Muscle

    c. The liver or stomach

    d. Adipose tissue

18. During auscultation, the bell of the stethoscope must not be placed too firmly on the skin because:

    a. This may cause the child to become uncooperative with the exam

    b. The skin will stretch, causing the bell to act like a diaphragm

    c. This will cause extraneous room noise to be heard more easily

    d. This affects the stethoscope earpiece alignment

19. A 17-year-old adolescent girl is at the clinic for an annual physical. Both her resting pulse and respirations are elevated. Her body temperature, blood pressure, and weight are within normal limits. She has no history of any cardiac or respiratory conditions. Which of the following may be a cause of her tachycardia and tachypnea?

    a. She is a regular runner and runs 3 miles a day

    b. She is on antidepressants

    c. She drinks six cups of coffee a day

    d. She takes biotin supplements

20. All of the following can cause a toddler to be flushed *except*:

  a. Fever
  b. Crying
  c. Increased physical activity
  d. Hypothyroidism

SAMPLE DOCUMENTATION: INTRODUCTION TO PHYSICAL ASSESSMENT

Write-Up Instructions

The following documentation template illustrates a sample pediatric general survey, which is the beginning of the physical examination. Subsequent chapters discuss each body system individually.

1. For each age group, infancy through adolescence, complete the following write-up template.
2. After completing each write-up, summarize the write-up in a paragraph.

Patient Name _____ Date of Birth _____ Date_____
Gender_____

Physical Examination

General Survey

1. General appearance_____
2. Level of consciousness_____
3. Facies_____
4. Position, posture, gait, mobility_____
5. Hygiene_____
6. Nutritional status_____
7. Behavior_____
8. Development_____

Vital Signs

1. Temperature (include route)_____
2. Heart rate (include site where assessed, e.g., apical, radial)_____
3. Respirations_____
4. Blood pressure (age ≥ 3 years)_____

Anthropometric Measurements

1. Weight (pounds and kilograms)_____ lbs _____kg
2. Height (length if age ≤ 2 years) _____ft/in. _____cm
3. Head circumference (age ≤ 3 years) _____in. _____cm
4. Body mass index (BMI) (≥ 2 years) include percentile_____

The Health Supervision Visit: Wellness Examinations in Children

CHAPTER OVERVIEW

A crucial element of pediatric health assessment is health supervision. This involves the determination of a child's physical and psychosocial health and wellness, assessment of parent or caregiver knowledge base, the delivery of clinical preventive services, and age-appropriate anticipatory guidance. This chapter helps the student refine skills in conducting the pediatric health supervision visit.

Expected Learning Outcomes

After reading Chiocca, *Advanced Pediatric Assessment, Second Edition*, Chapter 9, the learner will be able to:

1. Define the concept of a "medical home" and discuss its importance in the context of pediatric health care
2. Define "primary care" and discuss why it is critical to the delivery of quality pediatric health care
3. Discuss the timing of pediatric health supervision visits and the components of each visit

Essential Terminology

Access to care—having a regular source of comprehensive health care without barriers to services

Anticipatory guidance—health teaching provided at each well-child, health supervision visit. It educates the parents or caregivers about their child's next stage of physical and psychosocial development so that they know what to expect

Episodic care—care provided for a particular problem or complaint; no ongoing relationship is established between the patient and provider

Health screening—assessment aimed at identifying the potential for or early stages of a potential physical, psychosocial, or developmental problem; examples include developmental, newborn, lipid, hearing, vision, or depression screening

Health supervision visit—the primary health care visit that is done according to the American Academy of Pediatrics (AAP) periodicity schedule

Medical home—a model of delivering primary care that is accessible, continuous, comprehensive, family-centered, coordinated, compassionate, and culturally effective (AAP, 2008, p. 184)

Periodicity schedule—the AAP summary of the timing of recommendations for the history and physical examination, measurements, developmental assessment, preventive screening, immunizations, and anticipatory guidance for each well-child visit

Primary care—the provision of health promotion, disease prevention, health maintenance, patient education, diagnosis and treatment of acute and chronic illnesses in the context of a medical home

CRITICAL THINKING EXERCISES

Short-Answer Critical Thinking Exercises

1. Discuss what is meant by the term *medical home.*
2. To what does the term "new morbidity" refer when discussing health and illness in children?
3. Discuss why the timing of health maintenance visits to coincide with the recommended immunization schedule for children may actually decrease attendance at well-child health maintenance visits.
4. What are the basic components of the pediatric health supervision visit?
5. What is meant by the term *access to care?*
6. What is the "periodicity schedule?"
7. What are the *Bright Futures* health promotion themes?
8. What is anticipatory guidance? Why does it differ for each age group? Can it differ from child to child within an age group?
9. What are the AAP recommendations for health screening in children, from birth to age 21?

Critical Thinking Case Study Exercises

Exercise 1

List three anticipatory guidance topics in each of these boxes:

AGE GROUP	NUTRITION	ELIMINATION	SAFETY	SLEEP	GROWTH AND DEVELOPMENT
Infant					
Toddler					
Preschooler					
School-aged child					
Adolescent					

Exercise 2

Ariana is a 5-year-old girl who is brought to the clinic by her grandparents, who are her permanent guardians. She needs a kindergarten physical. Her grandparents state that they have her "baby shot" record with them. As you begin the physical, Ariana's grandfather says that she is a very picky eater, and he would like to know how he can get her to eat more fruits and vegetables, and eat a wider variety of foods.

1. What are the specific components of the health history that you should obtain for this particular child?
2. For a child of this age, what are the "do not miss" parts of the physical examination?
3. What screening does Ariana need? Are any lab tests needed?
4. According the AAP immunization schedule, is Ariana due for any immunizations?
5. What should the anticipatory guidance focus on? How will you answer the grandfather's questions?

Exercise 3

Trevor is a 16-year-old boy who is in the office for his annual physical examination. You need to gather the psychosocial history, and decide to use the BIHEADSS acronym as a guide:

BI = Body image
H = Home situation
E = Education or school performance
A = Activities
D = Drugs or dating patterns
S = Sexuality
S = Safety, suicidal ideation, or depression

1. What questions would you ask for each assessment category?

Exercise 4

Noah is a 9-month-old infant in the office for his health maintenance exam. He has been receiving well-child care at the same practice since birth. His prenatal, birth, and neonatal histories are unremarkable except for hyperbilirubinemia on day 3 of life.

1. What information needs to be gathered for the interval history?
2. What should the physical examination focus on?
3. Are there any maternal–infant assessments that should be made? If so, what are they?
4. What immunizations are due, if any?
5. What screening is due, if any?
6. What anticipatory guidance topics should be discussed at the end of the visit?

REVIEW QUESTIONS

1. Pediatric health supervision visits are an example of:

   a. Mortality prevention
   b. Primary prevention
   c. Morbidity prevention
   d. Secondary prevention

2. In a child without any eye or vision complaints, the first objective vision screening test is done at age:

   a. 1 year
   b. 2 years
   c. 3 years
   d. 4 years

3. A child has had a well-child examination and the following assessments have been made: weight, length, head circumference, cover/uncover test, gait, developmental screening, autism screening. This child is likely to be what age?

   a. 12 months
   b. 15 months
   c. 18 months
   d. 24 months

4. A child should have head circumference measured until age:

   a. 1 year
   b. 2 years
   c. 3 years
   d. 4 years

5. Newborns are screened for critical congenital heart disease. The timing of this screening is as follows:

   a. After 24 hours of age, before discharge from the hospital
   b. Any time before discharge
   c. Immediately after birth
   d. Within 24 hours of birth

6. A health maintenance examination is conducted on an 18-month-old child without any significant past medical history. Which of the following findings necessitates further action?

   a. The child has received only one MMR vaccine
   b. The child started walking independently just 4 months ago
   c. The child still drinks from a bottle
   d. The child says 20 words

7. Children should be screened for depression beginning at age:

   a. 9 years
   b. 11 years

    c. 13 years

    d. 15 years

8. The AAP recommends which of the following assessment tools when screening for alcohol or drug use?

    a. The CAGE questionnaire

    b. The Michigan Alcoholism Screening Test (MAST)

    c. The Alcohol Use Disorders Identification Test (AUDIT)

    d. The CRAFFT screening questionnaire

9. A normal, healthy full-term infant should be screened for iron deficiency anemia at age:

    a. 6 months

    b. 9 months

    c. 12 months

    d. 15 months

10. Of the following, which is the most *critical* physical assessment to make when conducting a sports physical (preparticipation examination)?

    a. Determination that the child has 20/20 vision

    b. Determination that the child is not overweight or obese

    c. Assessment of the child's immunization history

    d. Conduction of maneuvers to screen for hypertrophic cardiomyopathy

11. The following nutritional history is conducted: "Does your child drink from a bottle or sippy cup? Do you brush her teeth? Does she still use a pacifier? What kind of milk does she drink? How much juice does she drink?" This represents a nutritional history for which age group?

    a. Infant

    b. Toddler

    c. Preschooler

    d. School-aged child

12. The body mass index (BMI) measurement should be calculated and documented beginning at what age?

    a. 2 years

    b. 3 years

    c. 4 years

    d. 5 years

13. Which of the following topics would not be appropriate to include when providing anticipatory guidance to the parents of a 2-month-old?

    a. Sleep position

    b. Temper tantrums

    c. Starting the cup

    d. Introduction of solids

14. Which of the following anticipatory guidance topics should be discussed with the parents of a 3-year-old?

    a. Increasing fears
    b. Increasing temper tantrums
    c. Stranger anxiety
    d. Toilet training

15. Which of the following adolescent girls should receive a routine cervical dysplasia screening?

    a. A 17-year-old girl with complaints of dysmenorrhea
    b. A 14-year-old girl who just reached menarche
    c. A healthy 18-year-old
    d. Routine cervical dysplasia screening is not recommended until age 21 years

16. Anticipatory guidance for the parents of an 8-year-old girl should include:

    a. Preparation for puberty
    b. Increasing speech and language development
    c. Preparation for increased fears and imagination
    d. Information about contraception

17. Which of the following is an example of an essential physical assessment to make on an infant?

    a. Assessment for hip click
    b. Assessment of gait
    c. Assessment of BMI
    d. Assessment of the cover/uncover test

18. Which of the following is an example of an essential physical assessment to make on an adolescent?

    a. Forward bending test to screen for scoliosis
    b. Assessment of fine motor skills
    c. Assessment for metatarsus adductus
    d. Assessment of speech

19. The primary care provider is running 90 minutes behind schedule and is trying to prioritize anticipatory guidance teaching topics for an 18-month-old toddler whose weight, head circumference, and length are in the 75th percentile. In addition, toilet training has just begun, the child still takes two naps, and there are no developmental or behavioral concerns. Which of the following anticipatory guidance topics takes priority?

    a. Sleep
    b. Safety
    c. Nutrition
    d. Toilet training

20. An 11-year-old girl, Juliana, comes to the clinic for a health maintenance visit accompanied by her mother. The child and mother deny any complaints. Juliana gets As and Bs in school and has a best friend. Her physical exam is within normal limits. What screening, lab tests, or immunizations should Juliana have at this visit?

    a. Objective vision and hearing screening, sexually transmitted disease (STD) screen, pelvic exam, and screening for cervical dysplasia
    b. Depression screen, objective vision and hearing screening, primary measles vaccine
    c. Pneumococcal vaccine, cholesterol screening, depression screen
    d. Depression screen, cholesterol screening (if not done since age 9 years); Tdap, HPV, meningococcal, and annual flu vaccines

REFERENCE

American Academy of Pediatrics. (2008). Statement of reaffirmation: The medical home. *Pediatrics*, *122*(2), 450. doi:10.1542/peds.2008–1427

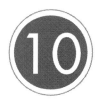

Assessment of Nutritional Status

CHAPTER OVERVIEW

This chapter focuses on the nutritional history for each age group, the areas of physical assessment that indicate a pediatric patient's nutritional status, and the accurate documentation of historical and physical findings.

Expected Learning Outcomes

After reading Chiocca, *Advanced Pediatric Assessment, Second Edition,* Chapter 10, the learner will be able to:

1. Obtain a thorough and accurate nutritional history for all pediatric age groups
2. Perform an age-appropriate physical assessment, focusing on nutritional status
3. Record all history and physical examination findings thoroughly and accurately

Essential Terminology

Acanthosis nigricans—a velvety, dark brown to black skin change found in skin folds and creases; a sign of insulin resistance

Anorexia—loss of appetite

Anthropometrics—measurements of body weight, height, and body proportions

Binge eating—consuming a large amount of food in a short amount of time

Body mass index (BMI)—measurement of the relationship between height and weight; calculated by dividing weight in kilograms (kg) by height in meters squared

Dysphgia—difficulty swallowing

Failure to thrive—the deceleration of height and weight growth in a child; growth parameters that decrease over two or more percentiles and are persistently below the third to fifth percentiles on the National Center for Health Statistics (NCHS) growth charts

Obesity—BMI equal to or greater than the 95th percentile on the NCHS growth charts

Overweight—BMI between the 85th and 95th percentile on the NCHS growth charts

Physiologic anorexia—decreased appetite related to slow body growth seen in the second year of life

Pica—craving and eating nonfood substances such as paper, dirt, hair, or sand

Purging—the conscious effort to control one's weight through self-induced vomiting, the use of laxatives, enemas, or diuretics

CRITICAL THINKING EXERCISES

Short-Answer Critical Thinking Exercises

1. Give examples of interview questions to ask when obtaining the nutritional history in children, from birth through adolescence.
2. Why do the questions asked during the nutritional history change for each age group? Be specific.
3. How is the child's social history relevant to his or her nutritional status? Give examples.
4. Are questions about a child's usual elimination or sleep patterns relevant to his or her nutritional assessment? Why or why not?
5. How can a child's weight affect his or her physical and psychosocial growth and development? Give examples for each age group.
6. What are the relevant components of the physical assessment when focusing on a child's overall nutritional status? Discuss each body system.
7. What body systems should be focused on during the physical assessment of an obese child or adolescent?
8. What is acanthosis nigricans, and what does it signify?
9. Why should an obese child or adolescent be assessed for wheezing? What other respiratory complications can occur in obese children and adolescents?
10. Discuss some musculoskeletal assessments that should be made in obese children and adolescents.
11. What are some maladaptive eating patterns in children? Give examples of some historical and physical findings that may be noted on routine well-child assessment.
12. What are some psychosocial complications of overweight and obesity in children and adolescents?
13. What are some medications that could affect a child's nutritional assessment?
14. What, if any, laboratory tests are part of the nutritional assessment?

Critical Thinking Case Study Exercises

Exercise 1

Alejandro is a 13-year-old Hispanic teen who comes to the clinic for an annual health maintenance visit. He is new to the practice, so his previous history is unknown. His vital signs and anthropometric measurements are as follows:

Temperature: 98.7 F
Pulse: 78
Respiratory rate: 16
Blood pressure: 144/88
Weight: 229 pounds (104 kg)
Height: 65 inches (172.7 cm)

1. What is Alejandro's BMI? Where does his BMI fall on the NCHS growth charts?
2. What specific parts of Alejandro's health history are important to know?
3. What information should be gathered in the following areas of the health history?
   a. Nutrition
      i. Dietary history
      ii. Weight changes
      iii. Gastrointestinal symptoms
   b. Elimination
   c. Social
   d. Sleep
   e. Developmental
   f. Review of systems
   g. Past medical history
   h. Past surgical history
   i. Family history
   j. Medications
4. What specific physical assessments are important to obtain on Alejandro, given the objective data listed here?

Exercise 2

Janelle is an 18-month-old toddler. Janelle's mother tells the provider that Janelle "loves milk," and drinks about eight to ten 8-ounce bottles of 2% cow's milk per day. She also drinks five to six 8-ounce bottles of apple juice each day. Her mother has not yet introduced the cup. When asked about solids, she states that Janelle is very picky and "doesn't eat much." On the NCHS growth charts for age and gender, Janelle's weight is in the 90th percentile, her length, the 50th percentile, and head circumference, 50th percentile.

1. What other historical data are important to know about Janelle that are not included here?
2. Given this information, what specific physical assessments are important to obtain on Janelle?
3. Is a developmental assessment especially important for Janelle? Why or why not?
4. Why is it important to obtain Janelle's social history?
5. How can Janelle's "picky" eating be interpreted? Give more than one answer.

Exercise 3

Michael is a 15-month-old toddler presenting for a health maintenance visit. This is his first well-child visit since age 6 months; all his other health care visits have been for acute health care issues. During the nutritional history, the provider learns that Michael has been drinking 2% cow's milk since age 8 months.

1. What other historical information should the provider obtain?
2. What should the provider focus on when measuring Michael's weight, length, and head circumference?
3. What specific physical assessments should the provider be sure to obtain?
4. What specific laboratory tests, if any, should be obtained?

Exercise 4

Julia is a 16-year-old adolescent. She is a gymnast who presents to the clinic in need of a sports physical. Julia's height is 65.5 inches, and her weight is 108 pounds. As soon as the medical assistant weighs her, Julia asks what she weighs. When told the amount, she looks upset and becomes quiet and withdrawn for the rest of the health care encounter.

1. What other historical information should the provider obtain?
2. What specific physical assessments are important to obtain on Julia?
3. What psychosocial assessments should be made?
4. What specific laboratory tests, if any, should be obtained?

REVIEW QUESTIONS

1. Which of the following subjective findings in the nutritional assessment of a 4-month-old should concern the health care provider?

   a. The mother uses tap water to mix the formula
   b. The mother breastfeeds and supplements with 20-calorie, ready-to-feed formula
   c. The mother has introduced solid food
   d. The mother feeds the infant on demand and not on a schedule

2. A nutritional assessment of a toddler should include all of the following *except*:

   a. Assessment of the type and amount of milk consumed per day
   b. Assessment of the type and amount of juice consumed per day
   c. Assessment of whether the child is still bottle-feeding
   d. Assessment of whether or not the toddler naps after eating

3. Which of the following subjective findings in the nutritional assessment of a 4-year-old is of concern to the pediatric health care provider?

   a. The child drinks 4 to 6 ounces of juice per day
   b. The child will only eat two different types of fruit and one vegetable
   c. The child drinks one 12-ounce can of soda roughly 5 days a week
   d. The child is a picky eater

4. During the nutritional assessment of a school-aged child, the provider should ask the child about all of the following *except*:

   a. What types of snacks the child consumes
   b. What the child drinks when thirsty

    c. If the child watches television while eating

    d. Whether the child thinks the family has enough money for food

5. During the nutritional assessment of an adolescent, the provider must be sure to inquire about:

    a. Whether the teen eats green vegetables

    b. Whether the teen drinks skim versus 2% milk

    c. Meal skipping

    d. Amount of meat consumption

6. Which of the following dietary factors would *most* likely be the major cause of iron deficiency anemia in a 15-month-old toddler?

    a. Refusal of fruits and vegetables

    b. Excessive cow's milk intake

    c. Consumption of 8 to 12 ounces of fruit juice per day

    d. Refusal of leafy green vegetables

7. Children at risk of malnutrition include all of the following *except*:

    a. A 6-month-old infant who drinks soy formula

    b. Children living in poverty

    c. Children with chronic illnesses

    d. A hospitalized child

8. Overweight children and adolescents should routinely be screened for:

    a. Hypertension

    b. Anemia

    c. Hyperthyroidism

    d. Hypoglycemia

9. When obtaining the nutrition-focused medical history, at what point is the presence of daily, persistent gastrointestinal symptoms considered severe?

    a. Five days

    b. One week

    c. Ten days

    d. Two weeks

10. Obesity in a child or adolescent may cause any of the following musculoskeletal findings *except*:

    a. Blount's disease

    b. Growth deceleration

    c. Flat feet

    d. Slipped capital femoral epiphysis

11. In a term infant, routine screening for iron deficiency anemia takes place between:

    a. 4 and 6 months of age

    b. 6 and 9 months of age

    c. 9 and 12 months of age

    d. 12 and 15 months of age

12. Assessment findings caused by iron deficiency anemia in a toddler may include all of the following *except*:

    a. Tooth decay

    b. Pale conjunctivae

    c. Overweight

    d. Pallor

13. Which of the following may be an objective finding in an adolescent girl with anorexia nervosa?

    a. Acanthosis nigricans

    b. Amenorrhea

    c. Binge eating

    d. Fatty liver disease

14. All of the following integumentary findings may be indicative of a nutritional problem *except*:

    a. Shiny mucous membranes

    b. Dry hair

    c. Purpura

    d. Alopecia

15. A mother reports that her toddler seems to have a sluggish appetite. This is within normal limits due to:

    a. Supplementing breastfeeding with formula for the first year of life

    b. Exclusive breastfeeding for the first year of life

    c. The age at which solid food was introduced into the child's diet

    d. The effects of physiologic anorexia

16. Acanthosis nigricans is most likely to be found with which of the following alterations in nutritional status?

    a. Iron deficiency anemia

    b. Protein deficiency

    c. Obesity

    d. Marasmus

17. Signs of protein-energy depletion in children include all of the following *except*:

    a. Ascites

    b. Edema

    c. Stomatitis

    d. Muscle wasting

18. A clinical manifestation found in kwashiorkor is:

    a. Loss of body fat

    b. Generalized edema

    c. Elevated serum albumin levels
    d. Hyperactivity

19. A clinical manifestation found in marasmus is:

    a. Stunted linear growth
    b. Near-normal weight
    c. Pedal edema
    d. Elevated serum albumin levels

20. Which of the following historical assessment findings obtained on a 6-month-old child is concerning and necessitates parental teaching?

    a. The mother breastfeeds and supplements with formula three times per day
    b. The mother has stopped breastfeeding because she has returned to work
    c. The parents give the infant one teaspoon of honey as needed for constipation
    d. The parents have started giving the infant small amounts of breast milk or formula in a cup

SAMPLE DOCUMENTATION: NUTRITIONAL ASSESSMENT

Patient Name _____ Date of Birth_____ Date_____
Gender_____

I. **Health History**
  A. **Reason for Seeking Health Care** (e.g., routine well-child examination; nutritional complaint)
  B. **Past Medical History**
    1. Prenatal, birth, neonatal histories
    2. Chronic health conditions
    3. Past hospitalizations
    4. Surgical history
    5. Family medical history
    6. Current medications
    7. Food allergies
    8. Review of systems
  C. **Nutritional History** (see *Advanced Pediatric Assessment, Second Edition*, Chapter 10, for age-specific assessment questions)
  D. **Elimination Patterns**
  E. **Dental History**
  F. **Developmental History**
  G. **Social History**

II. **Physical Examination**
  A. **Vital Signs**
  B. **Anthropometric Measurements**
    1. Weight
    2. Length/height
    3. Head circumference (age 3 years and younger)

      4. Weight for length/height
      5. BMI (age 2 years and older)
      6. Plot all measurements on growth charts
   C. **General**
      1. Behavior assessment
      2. Affect
      3. Emaciated or malnourished appearance
      4. Overweight/obesity
      5. Hygiene
   D. **Integumentary Assessment**
      1. Skin
         a. Edema
         b. Turgor
         c. Pallor
         d. Wound healing
      2. Hair
      3. Nails
      4. Acanthosis nigricans
   E. **Mouth**
      1. Lips
      2. Mucous membranes, oral cavity
      3. Gums
      4. Teeth
   F. **Eyes**
   G. **Musculoskeletal Assessment**
   H. **Neurologic Assessment**
   I. **Gastrointestinal Assessment**
   J. **Developmental Assessment**

NUTRITION ASSESSMENT: WRITE-UP

Use the space provided here to document all subjective and objective findings using the SOAP rubric.

Subjective—(historical information; chief complaint; history of present illness)

_____

_____

Objective—(vital signs, physical examination findings, results of laboratory and other diagnostic tests)

_____

_____

Assessment—(diagnosis [use ICD-10 codes]; other health issues that are identified)

_____

_____

Plan—(treatment, medications, therapies, teaching, referrals, follow-up care)

_____

_____

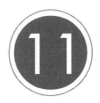

Assessment of the Neonate

CHAPTER OVERVIEW

The neonatal period is a time of numerous physical changes that occur during the transition from intrauterine to extrauterine life. Excellent history-taking and physical assessment skills are necessary for early recognition of existing or potential problems. This chapter helps the pediatric health care provider gain further understanding of gestational age assessment, the comprehensive neonatal history and physical examination, neonatal screening, and identification of at-risk infants.

Expected Learning Outcomes

After reading Chiocca, *Advanced Pediatric Assessment, Second Edition,* Chapter 11, the learner will be able to:

1. Obtain and interpret relevant prenatal, perinatal, and neonatal historical findings
2. Using a systematic approach, conduct a head-to-toe physical assessment of a neonate
3. Identify normal and abnormal anatomic and physiologic findings of the neonatal assessment
4. Describe methods of determining gestational age
5. Discuss classification of neonates by birth weight and gestational age
6. Demonstrate the ability to record all health assessment findings accurately and completely

Essential Terminology

Acrocyanosis—cyanosis of the hands and feet in the newborn; may be caused by cool ambient room temperatures, vasoconstriction, or hypoxemia; within normal limits in immediate neonatal period

Apgar score—a quantitative assessment of a neonate's cardiorespiratory function at birth; the Apgar score ranges from 0 to 10; score is done at 1 and 5 minutes of age and every 5 minutes until the score is 7 or greater; a low 5-minute Apgar score is associated with poor neurologic outcomes

Appropriate for gestational age (AGA)—neonatal weight between the 10th and 90th percentile for gestational age

Caput succedaneum—edema of the neonate's scalp caused by vaginal delivery and being pushed through the birth canal; more prominent in infants born to primiparous mothers; the edema crosses suture lines and resolves spontaneously in a few days

Cephalohematoma—a collection of blood between the periosteum and skull; does not cross suture lines; caused by prolonged second stage labor or vigorous use of surgical instruments (e.g., forceps) during vaginal delivery; may cause hyperbilirubinemia or anemia in the neonate; can take weeks to resolve

Chronologic age—the time elapsed after birth; also postnatal age

Corrected age ("adjusted age")—the term used to gauge the correct developmental age of a child up to age 3 years who was born preterm; calculated by subtracting the number of weeks the child was born before 40 weeks gestation from the child's current chronological age

Diastasis recti—the visible gap between the abdominal rectus muscles that becomes more prominent when the infant cries; a normal variant

Full-term infant—an infant born between 38 and 42 weeks gestation

Gestational age—the age of a neonate as defined by the time elapsed between the first day of the mother's last normal menstrual period and the day of delivery

Grunting—expiratory sound made during forced expiration of a closed glottis; a natural form of peak end expiratory pressure; caused by carbon dioxide retention

Lanugo—fine hair that covers the body of the fetus; the amount and location of lanugo depends on gestational age, familial and racial differences, hormones, metabolic and nutritional influences

Large for gestational age (LGA)—neonatal weight above the 90th percentile for gestational age

Late preterm infant—an infant born between 35 and 37 weeks gestation

Meconium—the neonate's first stool; texture is thick and sticky; color is dark green; should be completely passed by 2 to 3 days after birth

Molding—temporary skull deformity caused by pressure on the neonatal head while passing through the narrow birth canal

Neonate—a newborn infant aged birth to 28 days

New Ballard Score—a set of neuromuscular and physical assessments used to determine neonatal gestational age

Newborn screening—the screening for certain medical conditions in the immediate newborn period; includes screening for selected metabolic and genetic disorders, hearing loss, and critical congenital heart defects

Period of reactivity—behavioral and physiologic changes in the normal newborn that occur in the first 10 hours of extrauterine life

Postnatal age—the number of days or weeks after birth

Postterm infant—an infant born after 42 weeks gestation

Preterm infant—an infant born before 37 weeks gestation

Primitive reflex—a reflex that originates in the brainstem and central nervous system (CNS); occurs in response to a specific stimulus; many disappear as the CNS matures; sometimes remain throughout life

Small for gestational age (SGA)—neonatal a weight below the 10th percentile for gestational age

Teratogen—an agent or factor that causes malformation of an embryo or fetus

Thermoregulation—the process by which the neonate maintains core body temperature

Vernix caseosa—a greasy, white or pale yellow material composed of sebaceous gland secretions and exfoliated skin cells; appears during the third trimester and decreases as the fetus nears term

CRITICAL THINKING EXERCISES

Short-Answer Critical Thinking Exercises

1. List and explain the components of the prenatal, perinatal, and neonatal histories.
2. What is meant by "corrected gestational age"? How does this affect future assessments and for what length of time?
3. What is the New Ballard Score?
4. What are some risk factors for preterm birth?
5. Why is neonatal thermoregulation so critical?
6. How can the maternal health history affect the neonate? Give specific examples.
7. What parts of the neonate's social history are particularly important and relevant?
8. In what order should the neonatal physical examination be conducted? Are there any factors that influence the sequencing of the physical examination? What should always be the first step of the physical examination?
9. Describe neonatal physiologic stability.
10. What are the periods of reactivity immediately after birth?
11. Discuss the sequence for neonatal physical assessment.
12. What are some common, benign integumentary findings in the neonate? What are some abnormal findings that would necessitate further investigation?
13. Compare and contrast cephalohematoma and caput succedaneum. Discuss the expected length of time of resolution and any expected complications.
14. Discuss normal and abnormal ophthalmoscopic findings in the neonate. Which findings are within normal limits, which conditions may resolve spontaneously? Which findings necessitate immediate referral?
15. When inspecting the external ear, why do abnormal findings necessitate thorough assessment of the renal system, especially if the abnormal findings are bilateral?
16. Why is it so critical to assess nasal patency in the neonate?
17. What is transient tachypnea of the newborn (TTN)? What condition must be ruled out that has a similar presentation to TTN?

18. Differentiate between innocent and pathologic murmurs in the neonate
19. Compare and contrast normal and abnormal findings of the genitourinary system for both males and females.
20. Compare and contrast normal and abnormal findings of the musculoskeletal system in the neonate. Name some essential assessments from a medico-legal standpoint.
21. Discuss the neonatal neurologic assessment. Include discussion of primitive reflexes.
22. For each body system, identify and discuss the *essential* physical assessment that must be made in the neonatal period.
23. What does the Neonatal Behavioral Assessment Scale describe? How can the results be used?

Critical Thinking Case Study Exercises

Exercise 1

Ava is a 2-week-old neonate in the office for her regular health maintenance examination. When the provider asks if the mother has any concerns, she says that when she changes Ava's diaper, sometimes she sees a small amount of blood in the front of the diaper and is wondering if the bleeding may be caused by any sort of reaction to the type of diaper wipes she is using. The mother has no other concerns. Ava's vital signs and weight are within normal limits, and her prenatal, perinatal, and neonatal histories are unremarkable.

1. What other historical data should the provider gather from Ava's mother?
2. What should the physical examination focus on?
3. What is the likely assessment finding, and is this within normal limits?
4. What should the provider tell Ava's mother?

Exercise 2

Henry is a 4-day-old infant who is brought to the clinic by his parents. He was discharged from the hospital at 48 hours of life after a normal, spontaneous vaginal delivery. His mother is G_1, P_1 with an unremarkable prenatal history. The family history is unremarkable. Today, Henry's parents are concerned that he "is beginning to look yellow."

1. What other historical data should the provider gather from Henry's medical record from the nursery?
2. What other historical questions should the provider ask Henry's parents?
3. What should the physical examination focus on?
4. Are any laboratory tests necessary?

Exercise 3

Lisa is a 3-week-old infant brought to the clinic by her mother and grandmother. Lisa's mother states that she noticed white spots in the baby's mouth which she assumed were breast milk. However, in the past 2 days, she saw visible white spots right before breastfeeding, and tried cleaning Lisa's mouth with a washcloth. The white spots did not come off and some bled when Lisa's mother rubbed them. Lisa had an unremarkable prenatal, perinatal, and neonatal course. Her current vital signs are within normal limits and her weight, length, and head circumference are all at the 50th percentile.

1. What other information should be gathered for the history of present illness?
2. Should any other areas of the body be included in the history and physical assessment in Lisa's case?
3. What should the physical assessment include?
4. What, if any, assessments should the health care provider make on Lisa's mother?

Exercise 4

Juan is a 1-week-old infant who was brought to the clinic by his parents because they believe he may be constipated. They are first-time parents, and are also very concerned because Juan failed the auditory brainstem response (ABR) test at birth. Juan's physical assessment is unremarkable. His current vital signs are within normal limits and his weight, length, and head circumference are all at the 25th percentile.

1. What questions should be included in Juan's nutritional history?
2. What questions should be included in Juan's elimination history? Is there any information from his neonatal history that may be potentially relevant, depending on current historical findings?
3. What should Juan's physical examination focus on?
4. When should Juan have a repeat ABR?

REVIEW QUESTIONS

1. At each well-child visit, the neonate's anterior and posterior fontanelles are inspected and palpated. The posterior fontanelle should be closed by age:

   a. 2 months
   b. 6 months
   c. 9 months
   d. 12 months

2. A 12-hour-old neonate has edema on the scalp that crosses the suture lines. This is:

   a. Cephalohematoma
   b. Caput succedaneum
   c. Molding
   d. Craniosynostosis

3. The corneal blink reflex disappears:

   a. Approximately 4 hours after birth
   b. At age 4 to 6 months
   c. After the child is walking
   d. Never

4. During general inspection of the neonate, the examiner notes that the left leg appears to have an extra gluteal fold when compared with the right leg. It is essential that the examiner follow up with all of the following assessments *except*:

   a. Spurling maneuver
   b. Galleazzi maneuver
   c. Ortolani maneuver
   d. Barlow maneuver

5. The eye examination of a neonate reveals an asymmetrical corneal light reflex (Hirschberg test). This finding is interpreted as:

   a. Normal and should resolve by 4 to 6 months
   b. Normal and should resolve by 10 to 12 months
   c. Abnormal and requires an ophthalmology referral
   d. A sign of neonatal blindness

6. Which of the following findings observed during the physical examination of a 2-week-old neonate is *abnormal*?

   a. Positive Babinski reflex
   b. No independent head control
   c. Talipes equinovarus
   d. Metatarsus adductus

7. Of the following, which assessment finding is most indicative of a full-term infant?

   a. Long lanugo present on the infant's back
   b. Incurving of the upper pinnae only
   c. Palpable breast tissue of 8 mm
   d. Transparent skin over the abdomen

8. A 2-week-old infant presents to the clinic for the recommended health supervision visit. All of the following findings on the physical examination are considered within normal limits *except*:

   a. Palpable, open posterior fontanelle
   b. A grade I–II systolic ejection murmur heard best at the upper left sternal border
   c. An ear pit anterior to the right pinna
   d. Resting heart rate of 90 bpm

9. An otherwise healthy 3-day-old infant has small, yellowish-white, 1-mm papules scattered in a transverse, linear distribution along the nasal groove. These lesions are most likely:

   a. Erythema toxicum
   b. Milia
   c. Cutis aplasia
   d. Telangiectatic nevi

10. Baby Z, aged 6 weeks, has a bright red raised rubbery lesion on the occiput. It has a sharply demarcated border and is 2 cm in diameter. This lesion is a:

    a. Capillary ("strawberry") hemangioma
    b. Port-wine stain
    c. Mongolian spot
    d. Cavernous hemangioma

11. Which of the following is *not* a characteristic of the type of lesion that Baby Z has?

    a. It is not present at birth
    b. Growth of this lesion usually stops at about 6 to 12 months of age
    c. The lesion is expected to completely resolve by age 5 to 7 years
    d. This lesion will continue to gradually grow for the first 12 to 15 months of Baby Z's life

12. Of the following assessment findings in the newborn, which is considered an abnormal finding?

    a. Disconjugate gaze
    b. Webbed neck
    c. Sebaceous cysts on gums
    d. Head lag

13. Most primitive reflexes in the newborn disappear by age:

    a. 2 to 3 months
    b. 4 to 6 months
    c. 6 to 8 months
    d. 8 to 10 months

14. Which of the following is true regarding mongolian spots?

    a. These lesions are often mistaken for bruising
    b. These birthmarks occur predominantly in Caucasian children
    c. These lesions are at high risk for becoming malignant
    d. The birthmarks are bright red in color

15. A 1-week-old infant exhibits three to four beats of bilateral ankle clonus. This assessment:

    a. Indicates likely perinatal hypoxic-ischemic insult
    b. Is within normal limits until approximately age 3 months
    c. Indicates cranial nerve damage
    d. Is a red flag for cerebral palsy

16. Weak or absent femoral pulses in the neonate are indicative of:

    a. Coarctation of the aorta
    b. Ventricular septal defect
    c. Normal transition from fetal circulation
    d. Atrial septal defect

17. The health care provider observes the respirations of a 4-hour-old full-term neonate and notes rapid, shallow breaths with two 10-second periods of apnea; then the respirations return to normal. This assessment:

   a. Represents respiratory distress
   b. Signifies likely amniotic fluid aspiration
   c. Represents periodic breathing, a normal variation in the first few hours of life
   d. Signifies likely meconuim aspiration

18. The neonate is predisposed to hypothermia because he or she:

   a. Does not shiver
   b. Has decreased brown fat metabolism
   c. Has an immature liver
   d. Has a decreased body surface area

19. The following clinical presentation is *abnormal* during the neonatal transition period:

   a. Facial bruising and petechiae following a rapid delivery
   b. Respiratory rate of 68 and expiratory grunting
   c. Cranial molding in a vaginally delivered infant
   d. Heart rate of 180 during crying

20. At a corrected gestational age of 10 weeks, which of the following physical findings is within normal limits for an infant who was born at 32 weeks gestation?

   a. Abundant lanugo
   b. Skin that is translucent, smooth, and shiny
   c. Distinct creases extending across the entire palms of the hands
   d. Dolichocephaly

SAMPLE DOCUMENTATION: ASSESSMENT OF THE NEONATE

Name _____ Date of Birth _____ Date _____
Gender_____

I. **Health History**
   A. **Past Medical History**
      1. Prenatal history (see Table 6.2 of *Advanced Pediatric Assessment, Second Edition*)
      2. Birth history (see Table 6.2 of *Advanced Pediatric Assessment, Second Edition*)
      3. Neonatal history (see Table 6.2 of *Advanced Pediatric Assessment, Second Edition*)
         a. Prematurity
         b. Birth defects
         c. Cardiac conditions
         d. Respiratory conditions
         e. Genetic conditions
         f. Inborn errors of metabolism

4. Review of systems
5. Surgical history
6. Family medical history
7. Medications
8. Immunization status (hepatitis B)
9. Social history

II. **Physical Examination**
   A. **Vital Signs**
      1. Temperature
      2. Heart rate
      3. Respiratory rate
      4. Blood pressure (upper and lower extremity)
   B. **Anthropometric Measurements**
      1. Weight
      2. Length
      3. Head circumference
      4. Plot all measurements on growth charts
   C. **Integumentary Assessment**
      1. Inspect
         a. Color
         b. Perfusion
         c. Rashes
      2. Palpate
         a. Perfusion
         b. Capillary refill
   D. **Head**
      1. Inspect
         a. Shape and size
         b. Skull
         c. Scalp injuries
         d. Hair whorls
         e. Face
            i. Symmetry
            ii. Edema
            iii. Deformities
      2. Palpate
         a. Fontanelles
         b. Edema
         c. Cranial sutures
   E. **Eyes**
      1. Inspect
         a. Size, shape, position
         b. Coordination of eye movements
         c. Gaze
         d. Conjunctivae
         e. Sclerae
      2. Ophthalmoscopic examination
         1. Red reflex
         2. White reflex
         3. Symmetry of light reflex

F. Ears
   1. Inspect
      a. Pinna deformities
      b. Pinna placement
      c. Ear pits
      d. Skin tags
   2. Hearing assessment
      a. Startle response
      b. Evoked otoacoustic emissions or auditory brainstem response

G. Nose
   1. Inspect
      a. Nasal patency
      b. Nasal flaring
      c. Shape and placement
      d. Deformities

H. Oral Cavity
   1. Inspect
      a. Size and symmetry of lips
      b. Epstein pearls
      c. Natal teeth
      d. Tongue size
      e. Cleft lip/palate
      f. Excessive salivation
   2. Palpate
      a. Natal teeth

I. Neck
   1. Inspect
      a. Masses
      b. Movement
      c. Webbing
   2. Palpate
      a. Masses
      b. Lymph nodes

J. Chest
   1. Inspect
      a. Shape
      b. Symmetry
      c. Respiratory effort
      d. Nipples
   2. Auscultate
      a. Lung sounds
      b. Heart sounds
   3. Palpate
      a. Clavicles
      b. Sternum
      c. Ribs

K. Cardiovascular
   1. Inspect
      a. Color (skin and mucous membranes)
      b. Edema

        c. Precordial activity

        d. Bounding pulses

    2. Palpate

        a. Perfusion

        b. Point of maximum impulse

        c. Peripheral pulses

        d. Liver

    3. Auscultate

        a. Heart rate

        b. Heart sounds

        c. Murmurs

        d. Blood pressure

L. Abdomen

    1. Inspect

        a. Shape

        b. Symmetry

        c. Distention

        d. Defects

        e. Umbilicus

    2. Auscultate

        a. Bowel sounds

    3. Palpate

        a. Abdominal tone

        b. Liver

        c. Hernias

            i. Umbilical

            ii. Inguinal

        d. Femoral pulses

M. Genitourinary Assessment

    1. Inspection

        a. Female genitalia

            i. Labia

            ii. Clitoris

            iii. Discharge

            iv. Bleeding

        b. Male genitalia

            i. Penis

            ii. Location of urethral opening

            iii. Scrotum

    2. Palpate

        a. Testicles

N. Musculoskeletal Assessment

    1. Inspect

        a. Range of motion/movement

        b. Digits

        c. Hips

        d. Legs

        e. Gluteal folds

        f. Feet

2. Maneuvers
   a. Ortolani/Barlow maneuver
   b. Galeazzi maneuver
O. Neurologic Assessment
   1. Inspect
      a. Tone
      b. Posture
   2. Reflexes
      a. Primitive
      b. Deep tendon reflexes
P. Behavior
   1. Sleep states
   2. Awake states
   3. Transitional states
Q. Screening results
   1. Metabolic and genetic conditions
   2. Hearing
   3. Blood pressure (upper and lower extremity)
R. Parent–Neonate Interaction
S. Signs of Maternal Postpartum Depression

ASSESSMENT OF THE NEONATE: WRITE-UP

Use the space provided here to document all subjective and objective findings using the SOAP rubric.

Subjective—(historical information; chief complaint; history of present illness)

_____

_____

Objective—(vital signs, physical examination findings, results of laboratory and other diagnostic tests)

_____

_____

Assessment—(diagnosis [use ICD-10 codes]; other health issues that are identified)

_____

_____

Plan—(treatment, medications, therapies, teaching, referrals, follow-up care)

_____

_____

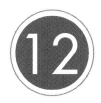

Assessment of the Integumentary System

CHAPTER OVERVIEW

Assessment of the integumentary system is an essential part of every pediatric health care visit. The condition of the skin, hair, and nails provides important information about both physical and emotional health. Many infectious diseases of childhood have cutaneous manifestations, and certain mental health illnesses may manifest as poor personal hygiene or self-injury. Child abuse and neglect may also produce a variety of clinical manifestations of the skin, hair, and nails related to intentional injury or poor nutritional status. This chapter helps the pediatric health care provider to gain further understanding of the child's developing integumentary system, and to recognize dermatologic clues to illness and injury.

Expected Learning Outcomes

After reading Chiocca, *Advanced Pediatric Assessment, Second Edition,* Chapter 12, the learner will be able to:

1. Explain the developmental considerations involving the integumentary system in infants and young children
2. Describe common pediatric primary and secondary skin lesions
3. Differentiate normal and abnormal physical findings of the skin, hair, and nails in the pediatric patient
4. Identify the physical and psychosocial illnesses that may have integumentary manifestations
5. Discuss how certain traditional grooming and healing practices affect pediatric integumentary assessment
6. Discuss skin and hair variations in dark-skinned children and how these affect integumentary assessment

Essential Terminology

Annular—ring-shaped

Atrophy—loss of epidermis or dermis; may cause thinning or depression of skin

Bulla—raised, fluid-filled lesion, greater than 1 cm in diameter

Confluent—lesions that run together

Contiguous—touching or adjacent

Crust—area of dried serum, blood, or exudate; may appear elevated; varies in color according to material that has dried at area

Cyanosis—bluish color to skin or mucous membranes caused by deoxygenated blood

Cyst—skin lesion that is raised, circumscribed, and encapsulated with a wall and lumen; filled with liquid or semi-solid material

Desquamation—skin peeling in sheets or scales

Discrete—lesions that are individual and distinct

Ecchymosis—macular or papular lesion greater than 10 mm in diameter caused by trauma to the area; blue, purple, yellow, green, or brown in color, depending on the age of the injury; does not blanch with pressure

Erosion—localized loss of epidermis; area often depressed, oozing, and moist and heals without scarring; does not extend into dermis

Erythema—redness of the skin due to capillary dilation; common etiologies include fever and inflammation

Excoriation—abrasion or hollowed-out area of epidermis, frequently caused by itching

Fissure—linear break in the skin extending into the epidermis and dermis

Hemangioma—a benign overgrowth of blood vessels in the dermis; lesion is often filed with blood; spontaneously involutes by age 5 to 7 years

Hematoma—accumulation of blood from ruptured blood vessel; bluish-red in color; greater than 1 cm in size

Iris—arranged in circles resembling a target

Jaundice—yellow color of skin and mucous membranes caused by elevated bilirubin levels in the blood

Keloid—benign overgrowth of skin of variable size that occurs after injury

Lichenification—thickened epidermis with visible furrows caused by chronic rubbing or scratching

Macule—discolored, circumscribed, nonpalpable, flat skin lesion, less than 1 cm in diameter

Nevus—well-circumscribed skin lesion caused by excess melanocytes; for example, mole

Nodule—firm, raised, solid lesion, greater than 1 cm in diameter

Pallor—pale, whitish skin color

Papule—raised, palpable, firm skin lesion, less than 1 cm in diameter

Patch—flat, nonpalpable discolored, irregularly shaped skin lesion, greater than 1 cm in diameter

Petechiae—pinpoint hemorrhages, dark red to purple in color, round and discrete, less than 2 mm in diameter

Plaque—raised, flat-topped superficial skin lesion, rough in texture, greater than 1 cm in diameter

Primary lesion—skin lesions that develop from previously normal skin

Pruritis—itchiness

Purpura—flat, dark red to purple lesions, 2 to 10 mm in diameter

Pustule—raised, superficial skin lesion, filled with purulent fluid

Scale—thin, exfoliated layers of epidermis

Scar—healed, fibrous tissue after dermal injury

Secondary lesion—skin lesions that evolve from primary lesions as a result of manipulation such as scratching, rubbing, or picking

Striae—pink or sliver bands, stripes, or lines on the skin caused by stretching

Telangiectasia—capillary dilation resulting in the appearance of small reddish-purple clusters

Tumor—raised, solid lesion; larger than a nodule

Ulcer—area of epidermis and dermis loss; varies in size; deeper than erosion

Vascular nevus (malformation)—overgrowth of blood vessels that occur during fetal development; can be flat, raised, or cavernous

Vesicle—superficially raised lesion containing serous fluid, less than 1 cm in size

Wheal—raised, irregular area of edema; solid, transient, and variable in size

Label the anatomic structures indicated on these illustrations.

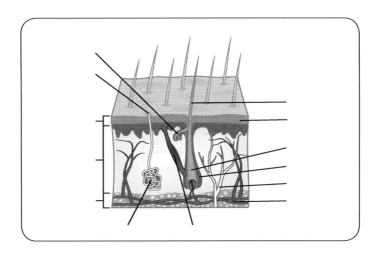

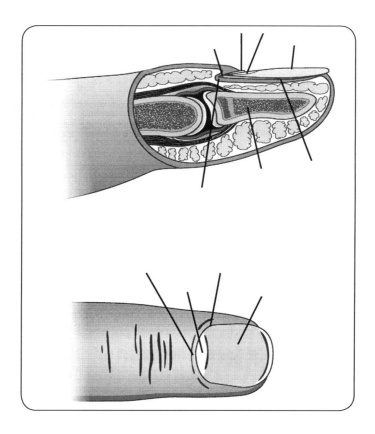

CRITICAL THINKING EXERCISES

Short-Answer Critical Thinking Exercises

1. Describe the main points of the integumentary assessment in a well child who presents for a health maintenance visit and is without complaints.
2. Inspection and palpation of the skin and hair provide information about a child's physical and emotional health. For each body system listed here, describe at least two integumentary findings that signal *physical* illness and the condition these findings may represent:

   a. Cardiovascular
   b. Respiratory
   c. Immunologic
   d. Neurologic
   e. Gastrointestinal
   f. Genitourinary
   g. Hematologic

3. What signs of *psychological* illness can be identified by examining a child's skin, hair, and nails?
4. Discuss how certain traditional grooming and healing practices influences pediatric integumentary assessment. Include discussion of how and why some of these practices may be confused with physical abuse or neglect,

and how the pediatric health care provider can distinguish normal and abnormal findings.

5. Discuss skin and hair variations in dark-skinned children and how these affect integumentary assessment. What are some normal variations? What are some cutaneous reaction patterns? Finally, what are some dermatologic conditions to which dark-skinned children are more prone?

Critical Thinking Case Study Exercises

Exercise 1

Matthew, a healthy 9-year-old Asian American boy, comes to the urgent care clinic complaining of a 2-week history of an intensely itchy scalp and rash on his neck. His mother states that several of his classmates at school have similar complaints. Close inspection of his scalp, hair, and neck reveals a maculopapular rash on the back of his neck with visible linear scratch marks, an erythematous scalp, and tiny, white specks on his hair.

1. What should the next assessment be in this situation?
2. What parts of Matthew's past medical history are important to know when formulating a differential diagnosis?
3. What is the most likely diagnosis, given the information above?
4. How will the provider make this diagnosis?

Exercise 2

Grace is a 2-year-old European American toddler whose family has just moved to the area, and she is new to the clinic. She is at the clinic for her annual health maintenance examination. The health care provider examining her skin notes dry, red papules on the extensor surfaces of all four extremities, and both cheeks are slightly erythematous with some evidence of mild lichenification. Her mother says that Grace has had this kind of rash on and off since she was about 3 months old and that when she has it, she scratches it until she bleeds.

1. What parts of Grace's medical and social history are important to know?
2. Is Grace's family history relevant to her current physical findings?
3. What other physical assessments should be made that would aid in confirming the diagnosis?
4. Based on this presentation, what is the differential diagnosis?
5. What is Grace's most likely diagnosis?
6. What teaching is important in order to prevent secondary infection of this condition?

Exercise 3

Jim, aged 15 years, presents to the school clinic with an erythematous, annular patch on both shins and knees. Jim has no significant past medical history and has no allergies. Jim is on the wrestling team.

1. What other historical questions would you ask Jim?
2. What should the physical examination focus on?

3. Based on Jim's history, and the description of his integumentary lesions, what condition do you suspect?

REVIEW QUESTIONS

1. The major function of the skin is to keep the body in homeostasis. This is achieved through all of the following *except*:

   a. Providing a protective barrier
   b. Vasoconstriction and vasodilation
   c. Excretion of toxins
   d. Vitamin A synthesis through the skin with exposure to sunlight

2. The *best* type of light in which to inspect a child's skin is:

   a. A well-lit examination room with neutral-colored walls
   b. Natural daylight
   c. A gooseneck lamp directed on the skin
   d. A fluorescent lamp

3. When obtaining the history specific to the integumentary system, which of the following age groups requires special tact and sensitivity due to the nature of certain skin conditions?

   a. Infants
   b. Toddlers
   c. Young school-aged children
   d. Older school-aged children and adolescents

4. When inspecting a child's skin during an annual health maintenance examination, which of the following is correct?

   a. Inspect only exposed areas in order to preserve privacy and modesty
   b. Inspect only areas of the skin that the examiner deems necessary
   c. Inspect only areas of the skin in which the child has a complaint
   d. Inspect the entire body, head to toe, beginning with the scalp and ending with the lower extremities

5. Which of the following dermatologic terms describes skin lesions that run together?

   a. Circinate
   b. Confluent
   c. Contiguous
   d. Guttate

6. An example of a primary skin lesion is:

   a. Atrophy
   b. Lichenification
   c. Nodule
   d. Crust

7. An example of a secondary skin lesion is:

   a. Desquamation
   b. Macule
   c. Patch
   d. Pustule

8. Palpation of the skin is done to assess all of the following *except*:

   a. Temperature
   b. Turgor
   c. Lesions
   d. Color

9. A raised, serous fluid-filled lesion, less than 1 cm in size is a:

   a. Bulla
   b. Vesicle
   c. Pustule
   d. Cyst

10. A nummular dermatologic arrangement can best be described as:

    a. Arranged in a line
    b. Having a stalk
    c. Coin-shaped
    d. Net-like

11. A 1-month-old has a pale pink macule on the right eyelid. This is likely a:

    a. Salmon patch ("stork bite")
    b. Capillary hemangioma ("strawberry mark")
    c. Nevus flammeus ("port-wine stain")
    d. Café-au-lait spot

12. Regarding the lesion in the previous question, the expected clinical outcome is:

    a. Does not enlarge or fade; may be associated with Sturge–Weber syndrome
    b. Usually involutes by age 5 to 7 years
    c. Benign but permanent
    d. Benign and fades with time, usually by age 1 year

13. When inspecting hair distribution in a child, thin hair may be due to all of the following *except*:

    a. Seborrhea
    b. Trictillomania
    c. Abuse or neglect
    d. Drug toxicity

14. A 10-year-old child presents for an annual physical examination. The child confirms daily fast food and soft drink consumption. The child's body mass index (BMI) is in the 99th percentile. Given this history, which of the following integumentary assessments is essential and relevant for this child?

a. Inspection for pityriasis alba
b. Inspection for acanthosis nigricans
c. Tzanck's smear
d. Wood's light examination

15. Which of the following dermatologic conditions is more common in dark-skinned children?

a. Pityriasis alba
b. Café-au-lait spots
c. Milia
d. Nevus flammeus

16. A 7-year-old child with a recent history of tinea corporis has a raised, boggy, tender, pustular mass on the scalp with localized alopecia. The most likely diagnosis is:

a. Alopecia areata
b. Traction alopecia
c. Kerion
d. Impetigo

17. Dark blue-purple, irregularly shaped macules, primarily seen in dark-skinned infants in the lumbosacral and gluteal areas are:

a. Café-au-lait spots
b. Congenital pigmented nevi
c. Cavernous hemangiomas
d. Mongolian spots

18. Regarding the lesion in the previous question, the expected clinical outcome is:

a. Benign and usually fades by age 5 to 7 years
b. Benign but permanent
c. Benign and fades with time, usually by age 1 year
d. Benign and fades with time, usually by puberty

19. A school-aged child has several honey-colored, thin-roofed vesicles on his upper lip and around his nares. This common skin condition is most likely:

a. Herpes simplex
b. Impetigo
c. Coxsackie virus
d. Acne

20. A 3-year-old child has a lesion on her trunk. It is a flat, scaly, erythematous circular patch with central clearing and raised borders. This common skin condition is most likely:

    a. Atopic dermatitis
    b. Folliculitis
    c. Contact dermatitis
    d. Tinea corporis

SAMPLE DOCUMENTATION: INTEGUMENTARY ASSESSMENT

Patient Name _____ Date of Birth _____ Date _____
Gender _____

  I. **Health History**
    A. Reason for Seeking Health Care (e.g., routine well-child examination; integumentary complaint)
      1. Past medical history
        a. Prenatal, birth, neonatal histories (e.g., syndromes)
        b. Chronic integumentary conditions (e.g., atopic dermatitis)
        c. Past hospitalizations related to integumentary system (e.g., burns, injuries or infections)
        d. Surgical history
        e. Family medical history (e.g., atopy)
        f. Current medications
        g. Social history (neglect; poor personal hygiene)
        h. Immunization history
        i. Review of systems
      2. Nutritional history (condition of skin)

  II. **Physical Examination**
    A. Assessment of General Appearance
    B. Inspect Skin
    C. Palpate Skin

ASSESSMENT OF THE INTEGUMENTARY SYSTEM: WRITE-UP

Use the space provided here to document all subjective and objective findings using the SOAP rubric.

Subjective—(historical information; chief complaint; history of present illness)

_____

_____

Objective—(vital signs, physical examination findings, results of laboratory and other diagnostic tests)

_____

_____

Assessment—(diagnosis [use ICD-10 codes]; other health issues that are identified)

_____

_____

Plan—(treatment, medications, therapies, teaching, referrals, follow-up care)

_____

_____

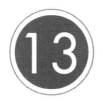

Assessment of the Head, Neck, and Regional Lymphatics

CHAPTER OVERVIEW

This chapter helps the pediatric health care provider to conduct an age- and developmentally appropriate examination of the head, neck, and lymph nodes; to recognize deviations from normal; and to accurately record assessment findings.

Expected Learning Outcomes

After reading Chiocca, *Advanced Pediatric Assessment, Second Edition*, Chapter 13, the learner will be able to:

1. Obtain a thorough and accurate history related to the head, neck, and lymph nodes in the pediatric patient
2. Accurately conduct an age- and developmentally appropriate physical examination of the head, neck, and lymph nodes in the pediatric patient and distinguish normal and abnormal findings
3. Analyze historical and physical assessment findings related to the head, neck, and lymph nodes, and use these data to make accurate assessments and diagnoses
4. Accurately record history and physical assessment findings related to assessment of the head, neck, and lymph nodes

Essential Terminology

Brachycephaly—occipital flattening; often caused by prolonged supine positioning

Caput succedaneum—localized subcutaneous edema over the presenting part of the scalp in a newborn; edema crosses the suture lines

Cephalocaudal—head-to-toe development; corresponds to the timing of myelination of the spinal cord and achievement of gross motor milestones

Cephalohematoma—swelling of the neonate's scalp caused by subperiosteal collection of blood; does not cross suture lines

Cranial molding—an abnormal shape of the head that is seen in neonates in the immediate postpartum period; caused by pressure exerted on the skull during delivery and is considered normal during the first 7 days of life

Cranial sutures—soft, fibrous tissue spaces that join the cranial bones

Craniosynostosis—premature closure at birth of one or more cranial sutures; sometimes known as craniostenosis

Craniotabes—a softening and thinning of the bones of the skull, assessed by palpation

Dolichocephaly—a condition in which the head is disproportionately long and narrow

Fontanelle—soft areas of the infant's skull that are formed when two or three cranial bones merge

Hydrocephaly—enlargement of the head due to increased intracranial pressure

Lymphadenopathy—lymph node tissue that measures greater than 1 cm in diameter; can be caused by infection, allergies, or neoplasm

Macewen's sign—resonant percussion sound heard when the surface of the parietal bone is tapped in an infant; in infants whose fontanels are still open, this is a normal finding; in older infants this may indicate increased intracranial pressure

Macrocephaly—occipital-frontal head circumference more than two standard deviations (SD) above the mean for age and sex, or one that is growing too rapidly

Microcephaly—occipital-frontal head circumference that is more than two SD below the mean for age and sex, or one that is not growing at the normal rate

Opisthotonos—extreme hyperextension of the neck

Plagiocephaly—flattening of the skull in one particular area; often due to prolonged positioning in one spot

Torticollis—injury to the sternocleidomastoid muscle that causes limited range of motion involving lateral movement of the neck

Lable the anatomic structures indicated on these illustrations.

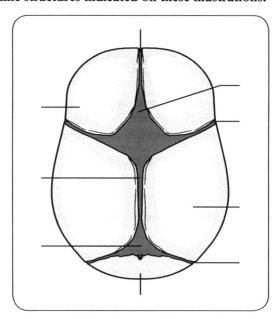

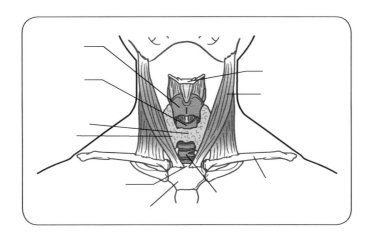

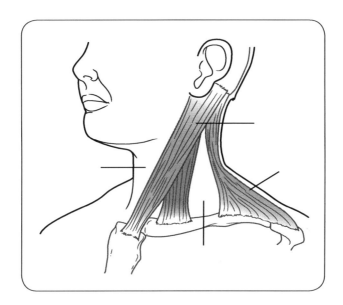

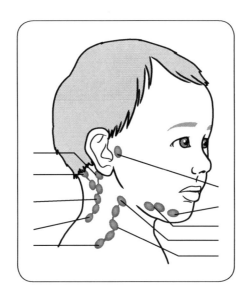

CRITICAL THINKING EXERCISES

Short-Answer Critical Thinking Exercises

1. Discuss the difference between caput succedaneum and cephalohematoma in the neonate.
2. Discuss normal and abnormal findings upon inspection and palpation of the anterior fontanelle.
3. When should the anterior fontanelle close? Why does the anterior fontanelle close later than the posterior fontanelle? What may cause a delay in closure of the anterior fontanelle?
4. At what age does a normal, healthy, full-term infant gain head control? What are possible causes of delay in achieving head control?
5. What are some causes of micro-/macrocephaly?
6. What is dolichocephaly? What causes it?
7. What is plagiocephaly? What causes it?
8. What is torticollis? What causes it?
9. Describe characteristics of lymph nodes that are within normal limits and those that are cause for concern.
10. What is meant by the term, "shotty" nodes? Is this a normal or abnormal finding?
11. Describe the process of palpation of the thyroid gland in a young child. At what age should the provider begin examining the thyroid in young children?

Critical Thinking Case Study Exercises

Exercise 1

Joshua is a healthy 6-month-old infant boy with occipital plagiocephaly and alopecia.

1. What historical questions should be asked?
2. Is Joshua's perinatal or neonatal history relevant?
3. What should the physical examination focus on?
4. What is the likely diagnosis?

Exercise 2

Pramod is a 5-year-old boy who was brought to the clinic with complaints of fever, cough, nasal congestion, and ear pain for 3 days. Currently, Pramod is febrile with a temperature of 101°; heart rate is 88; respiratory rate is 20; blood pressure is 88/58. He is in no respiratory distress and lung sounds are clear bilaterally. His nasal turbinates are erythematous with pale green drainage. Both tympanic membranes are pale pinkish-gray with visible landmarks. Anterior and posterior cervical lymph nodes are enlarged, soft, and moveable.

1. What elements of Pramod's history are important to know regarding his current complaints?
2. What other information should the health care provider gather about the history of present illness (HPI)?
3. What other objective assessments, if any, are necessary to obtain on Pramod? What should the physical examination focus on?

4. Given Pramod's age, are there any special considerations regarding physical examination techniques?
5. What is your assessment of Pramod's lymph nodes?
6. Is this finding within normal limits?

Exercise 3

Ramona is a 3-year-old girl who presents with low-grade fever that began 1 to 2 days before the onset of abdominal pain; a history of rash that is intensely pruritic; and signs and symptoms that include headache, malaise, anorexia, cough, and sore throat. Her physical examination reveals occipital lymphadenopathy.

1. What specific part of Ramona's history would you like to know?
2. What would you like to know about the characteristics of her rash?
3. What else should her physical examination include?
4. What condition do you suspect?

Exercise 4

During the physical examination of a 2-day-old infant girl, her neck is assessed.

1. State the steps in assessment of the neck in the newborn infant.
2. What are you looking for?
3. What are normal findings?
4. What are abnormal findings?

REVIEW QUESTIONS

1. At the 1-week visit, a newborn presents with edema of the scalp that crosses suture lines. This is:

   a. Cephalohematoma
   b. Intentional injury
   c. Hydrocephalus
   d. Caput succedaneum

2. A normal, healthy, full-term infant should achieve full and complete head control, with no head lag, by age:

   a. 2 months
   b. 4 months
   c. 6 months
   d. 9 months

3. The posterior fontanelle should close by age:

   a. 2 months
   b. 6 months
   c. 8 months
   d. 12 months

4. An anterior fontanelle that measures greater than 4 to 5 cm (2 in.) in diameter may be within normal limits, or it may indicate:

   a. Hyperthyroidism versus hypothyroidism
   b. Down syndrome
   c. Microcepahaly
   d. Craniotabes

5. Which of the following conditions can cause microcephaly in an infant?

   a. Tuberous sclerosis
   b. Neurofibromatosis
   c. Fetal alcohol syndrome
   d. Hyperpituitarism

6. Head and chest circumferences should be equal at:

   a. 6 months of age
   b. 1 year of age
   c. 2 years of age
   d. 3 years of age

7. The anterior fontanelle should close by:

   a. 2 to 3 months of age
   b. 6 to 9 months of age
   c. 12 to 18 months of age
   d. 18 to 24 months of age

8. Young infants may be prone to fungal or bacterial infections of the skin on the anterior neck because of:

   a. Their immature immune system
   b. Neck webbing that generally resolves by age 2 months
   c. Their limited neck range of motion that generally resolves by age 2 months
   d. Their short neck and folds of skin

9. Prominence of the frontal area of the cranium ("bossing") is seen with:

   a. Prematurity
   b. Hydrocephalus
   c. Dolichocephaly
   d. Craniosynostosis

10. The fontanelles are best inspected with infants or toddlers:

   a. Lying supine on the parent's lap
   b. Supine on the examination table
   c. Sitting upright on the parent's lap
   d. Lying prone on the examination table

11. A palpable, raised, tender, boggy mass with scattered pustules on the scalp is likely a:

    a. Kerion
    b. Lymphadenopathy
    c. Cephalohematoma
    d. Caput succedaneum

12. A healthy 1-week-old infant has limited range of motion with lateral movement of the neck. The examiner suspects:

    a. Opisthotonos
    b. Klippel–Feil syndrome
    c. Noonan syndrome
    d. Torticollis

13. The examiner is conducting a newborn exam on a healthy 2-day-old male infant and palpates a mobile, nontender, nonerythematous mass with a firm center. This finding is likely a(n):

    a. Thyroid tumor
    b. Fractured clavicle
    c. Cystic hygroma
    d. Enlarged parotid gland

14. Which of the following describes characteristics of lymph nodes that suggest malignancy?

    a. Small, firm, rubbery, nontender, mobile lymph nodes
    b. Enlarged, painful, soft and moveable nodes
    c. Painless lymph node that is hard and fixed to the underlying tissue
    d. Enlarged, firm, warm, and tender lymph node

15. The nurse practitioner is palpating a child's lymph nodes during the physical exam. The practitioner is aware that normal lymph nodes feel:

    a. Firm, warm, and tender
    b. Small, moveable, soft, and nontender
    c. Warm, tender, firm, freely moveable
    d. Hard, nontender, fixed, clumped

16. A child has occipital lymphadenopathy. Which of the following conditions should be suspected?

    a. Tinea capitis
    b. Stomatitis
    c. Streptococcal pharyngitis
    d. Infectious mononucleosis

17. Which of the following conditions must be considered when assessing a child with supraclavicular lymphadenopathy?

    a. Malignancy
    b. Oral and dental infections

    c. Infectious mononucleosis

    d. Postimmunization response

18. With the exception of the anterior cervical lymph nodes, lymphadenopathy is defined as lymph node tissue that measures:

    a. Greater than 0.5 cm in diameter

    b. Greater than 1 cm in diameter

    c. Greater than 1.5 cm in diameter

    d. Greater than 2 cm in diameter

19. Lymph tissue size is at its largest, approximately two times adult size, by age:

    a. 6 years

    b. 8 years

    c. 10 years

    d. 12 years

20. Lymph tissue begins to shrink, becoming adult sized beginning in:

    a. Late infancy

    b. Toddlerhood

    c. Early school age

    d. Early adolescence

SAMPLE DOCUMENTATION: ASSESSMENT OF THE HEAD, NECK, AND REGIONAL LYMPHATICS

Patient Name _____ Date of Birth_____ Date_____
Gender_____

I. **Health History**

  A. **Reason for Seeking Health Care** (e.g., routine well-child examination; complaint related to the head, neck, or lymph nodes)

    1. Past medical history

      a. Prenatal, birth, neonatal histories

      b. Chronic health conditions

      c. Past hospitalizations

      d. Surgical history

      e. Family medical history

      f. Current medications

      g. Immunization history

      h. Review of systems

    2. Developmental history

    3. Social history

II. Physical Examination
   A. Head
      1. Inspection of head
      2. Palpation
      3. Percussion
   B. Neck
      1. Inspection
      2. Palpation
      3. Auscultation
   C. Lymph Nodes
      1. Inspection
      2. Palpation

ASSESSMENT OF THE HEAD, NECK, AND REGIONAL LYMPHATICS: WRITE-UP

Use the space provided here to document all subjective and objective findings using the SOAP rubric.

Subjective—(historical information; chief complaint; history of present illness)

_____

_____

Objective—(vital signs, physical examination findings, results of laboratory and other diagnostic tests)

_____

_____

Assessment—(diagnosis [use ICD-10 codes]; other health issues that are identified)

_____

_____

Plan—(treatment, medications, therapies, teaching, referrals, follow-up care)

_____

_____

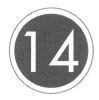

Assessment of the Ears

CHAPTER OVERVIEW

Assessment of the ears is an essential skill for the pediatric health care provider to possess. Important skills include obtaining a thorough history; an age-appropriate physical examination of the external ear, external auditory canal, and tympanic membrane; and the ability to perform an efficient and accurate otoscopic examination. Familiarity with age-appropriate receptive and expressive language milestones, and risk factors for and signs and symptoms of hearing loss are necessary for early identification of hearing loss in infants and children.

Expected Learning Outcomes

After reading Chiocca, *Advanced Pediatric Assessment, Second Edition,* Chapter 14, the learner will be able to:

1. Identify normal anatomic landmarks of the external and middle ear
2. Examine the external and middle ear and distinguish normal and abnormal findings
3. Identify normal and abnormal findings upon otoscopic inspection of the tympanic membrane
4. Analyze historical and physical assessment findings related to the ear and use these data to make accurate assessments and diagnoses
5. Discuss normal receptive and expressive language milestones in children, from birth through adolescence
6. Recognize risk factors for and signs of hearing loss in infants, children, and adolescents

Essential Terminology

Acute otitis media—a middle ear infection with viral or bacterial etiology; causes the tympanic membrane to become erythematous, with the contours and landmarks distorted as a result of fluid or purulent material accumulation behind the membrane

Cerumen—a sticky or flaky substance found in the external auditory canal, the function of which is to lubricate and clean the ear canal, trap dirt and other debris, and repel water from the tympanic membrane

Cochlea—the inner ear structure that contains the organ of Corti, the sensory organ for hearing

Concha—a hollow, bowl-like structure in the external ear that leads to the external auditory canal

Conductive hearing loss—hearing loss caused by blocked transmission of sound waves through the external auditory canal to the inner ear

Cone of light—a triangular-shaped light reflection seen when the otoscope light is reflected on the tympanic membrane

Eustachian tube—the structure that connects the middle ear to the nasopharynx; it has three main functions: (a) protection of the middle ear from excessive sound, pressure fluctuations, and secretions; (b) drainage of any middle ear secretions to the nasopharynx; and (c) equalization of pressure on both sides of the tympanic membrane

External auditory canal—the passageway that begins at the concha and ends at the tympanic membrane; its function is to funnel sound to the tympanic membrane

External ear—the cartilaginous outer part of the ear that is visible; its function is to collect sound inward. Comprises the pinna, external auditory canal, and tympanic membrane

Incus—the middle of the three ossicles; also known as the "anvil"

Inner ear—a fluid-filled structure located within the temporal bone; contains structures necessary for both hearing and balance

Malleus—the first of the three ossicles; also called the "hammer"; holds the tympanic membrane slightly inward, resulting in a concave shape; this is also what creates the cone of light

Middle ear—an air-filled space inside the temporal bone that contains the ossicles; connects to the eustachian tube and nasopharynx

Organ of Corti—the sensory organ for hearing; it contains auditory receptor hair cells that transmit impulses to the auditory nerve, then to the brain to be interpreted as sound

Ossicles—three tiny bones within the middle ear, consisting of the malleus (hammer), incus (anvil), and stapes (stirrup); these bones play a role in hearing by transmitting sounds to the inner ear

Otalgia—ear pain

Otitis media with effusion—the presence of mucoid or serous fluid behind the tympanic membrane, which often results in air bubbles visable behind the membrane and decreased mobility of the tympanic membrane on pneumatic otoscopy

Otorrhea—drainage from the ear

Pars flaccida—the upper, smaller, flexible, triangular portion of the tympanic membrane above the short process of the malleus

Pars tensa—the taut, larger portion of the tympanic membrane below the short process of the malleus

Pinna—also referred to as the auricle; the visible part of the ear seen outside the head

Pneumatic otoscopy—an assessment method to determine the mobility of the tympanic membrane using a small insufflation of air through a bulb apparatus attached to the otoscope; used to help diagnose acute otitis media and otitis media with effusion

Rinne test—a test conducted with a tuning fork to evaluate both conductive and sensorineural hearing by comparing air and bone conduction of sound when the vibrating tuning fork is placed on the mastoid process

Romberg test—a test of balance conducted to assess vestibular function

Semicircular canals—structures in the inner ear that play a role in maintaining equilibrium by detecting motion and balance

Sensorineural hearing loss—hearing loss caused by damage to the cochlea or auditory nerve fibers

Short process of the malleus—the part of the malleus that is visible through the tympanic membrane

Stapes—the innermost of the three ossicles; also known as the "stirrup"

Tinnitus—ringing in the ears

Tympanic membrane—an extremely thin, translucent, oval-shaped membrane that separates the outer ear from the middle ear

Umbo—the bottom portion of the malleus that is visible through the tympanic membrane

Vertigo—dizziness characterized by a spinning sensation

Vestibule—the inner ear structure that leads to the cochlea and semicircular canals and contains receptors necessary for the maintenance of equilibrium and balance

Weber test—a test conducted with a vibrating tuning fork to evaluate both conductive and sensorineural hearing; assessment is made to determine if sound is heard equally in both ears or is lateralized to one ear

Whisper test—a gross measurement of hearing acuity; conducted by asking the child to correctly repeat words spoken in a whisper; usually conducted on children aged 3 years and older

Label the anatomic structures indicated on these illustrations.

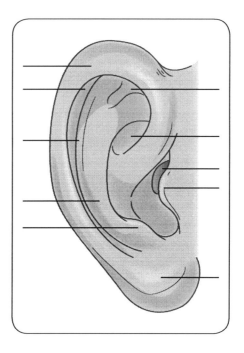

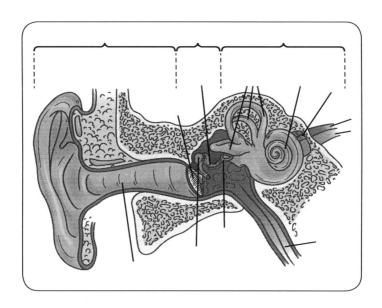

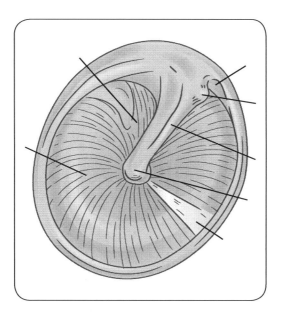

CRITICAL THINKING EXERCISES

Short-Answer Critical Thinking Exercises

1. Describe the assessment technique *pneumatic otoscopy*. What does pneumatic otoscopy assess? Discuss why this is an essential skill for the pediatric health care provider.
2. To complete the examination of the tympanic membrane in an infant or toddler, what must the pediatric health care provider consider in order to ensure safe and clear visualization of the tympanic membrane?
3. Compare and contrast the physical findings seen in the tympanic membrane of a child with acute otitis media and one with otitis media with effusion.
4. In what age group is hearing assessment most critical, and why?
5. Why are allergies a risk factor for developing acute otitis media and otitis media with effusion?

Critical Thinking Case Study Exercises

Exercise 1

Trevor is an 18-month-old African American boy who is brought to the clinic for an annual health maintenance visit. His prenatal, perinatal, and neonatal histories are unremarkable. Trevor is still bottle fed and has a history of three episodes of acute otitis media. His mother reports that he says about eight words, and that only she and his father can understand him. She also reports that he has trouble following simple directions and that temper tantrums have started. His length, weight, and head circumference are at the 50th percentile. Because he is 18 months of age, developmental screening is conducted.

1. What other parts of this child's medical history are important to know?
2. What developmental milestones should be assessed during Trevor's health visit?

3. Are Trevor's language milestones as indicated in the history within normal limits?
4. What specific language assessments should be conducted?
5. Does Trevor need any additional testing or assessments?

Exercise 2

Liliana is a 14-month-old Mexican American toddler whose mother brings her to the clinic with a 3-day history of fever, rhinorrhea, and cough. This morning, her mother reports that Liliana began tugging at her ear and has been very fussy. Liliana has a 3-year-old brother who began coughing this morning, but he is otherwise without complaints. Both Liliana and her brother attend day care 3 days per week. Currently, Liliana is sitting on her mother's lap crying and pulling on her right ear. She has a fever of 103°F (39.4°C), thick nasal discharge in both nares, and is coughing intermittently.

1. What aspects of Liliana's health history are important to know regarding her current complaints?
2. What other information should the health care provider gather about the history of present illness (HPI)?
3. What other objective assessments should be obtained on Liliana?
4. What should the physical examination focus on?
5. What is a specific physical examination technique that should be used in this instance?
6. Given Liliana's age, are there any special considerations regarding physical examination techniques?

REVIEW QUESTIONS

1. When determining the height of the pinna, the examiner draws an imaginary horizontal line from the outer canthus of the eye to the occiput. Which of the following describes a measurement that is within normal limits?

   a. The top of the pinna should meet or cross the imaginary horizontal line, deviating no more than 10 degrees from a line perpendicular to the horizontal line.
   b. The top of the pinna should meet or cross the imaginary horizontal line, deviating no more than 20 degrees from a line perpendicular to the horizontal line.
   c. The top of the pinna should be even with the outer canthus of the eye.
   d. The top of the pinna should be 1 cm above the outer canthus of the eye.

2. A 2-year-old girl presents to the clinic with fever, rhinorrhea, and ear pain and is diagnosed with her fourth episode of acute otitis media. When collecting the history, the health care provider should focus on all of the following elements *except:*

   a. History of breast versus bottle feeding
   b. History of secondhand smoke exposure

   c. History of expressive speech milestones
   d. History of co-sleeping after age 1 year

3. All of the following are risk factors for hearing loss in children aged 29 days to 2 years *except:*

   a. History of receiving extracorporeal membrane oxygenation
   b. Prenatal history of maternal chlamydia treated with azithromycin in the second trimester
   c. History of head trauma
   d. History of bacterial meningitis

4. The health care provider is inspecting the tympanic membrane of a 3-year-old child. Which of the following describes a normal finding?

   a. Pale light reflex
   b. Pale white tympanic membrane
   c. Pearly grey to light pink tympanic membrane
   d. Opaque tympanic membrane

5. The landmarks of the normal tympanic membrane should be easily visible upon inspection, including the cone of light reflex. Using the face of a clock as a reference point, at which position is this reflex visible on the *left* tympanic membrane?

   a. 1 o'clock
   b. 3 o'clock
   c. 5 o'clock
   d. 7 o'clock

6. Which of the following physical assessment techniques is used when acute otitis media or otitis media with effusion is suspected?

   a. Inspection of the tympanic membrane
   b. Pneumatic otoscopy
   c. Assessment of hearing delay
   d. Palpation of the tragus

7. Which of the following age groups is typically most resistant to the otoscopic examination?

   a. Neonates
   b. Young infants
   c. Older infants and toddlers
   d. Preschoolers

8. Which of the following anatomic differences place infants at greater risk for middle ear infections?

   a. Eustachian tube is longer and narrower
   b. Eustachian tube is shorter and wider

   c. Eustachian tube lies in a vertical plane

   d. Eustachian tube lies at a 90-degree angle

9. Which of the following describes the correct technique for optimal otoscopic visualization of the tympanic membrane in children aged 3 years and younger?

   a. Grasp the pinna and pull gently downward, outward, and backward, while directing the speculum upward

   b. Grasp the pinna and pull gently upward, backward, and slightly away from the head, while directing the speculum downward

   c. Grasp the pinna and pull gently outward and forward, while directing the speculum upward

   d. Grasp the pinna and pull gently outward, and forward, while directing the speculum downward

10. Inspection of the tympanic membrane during otoscopic examination reveals distorted anatomical landmarks and amber-colored bubbles behind the membrane. Pneumatic otoscopy reveals decreased movement. These findings most likely indicate:

   a. Acute otitis media

   b. Otitis externa

   c. Otitis media with effusion

   d. Tympanic membrane perforation

11. Which of the following types of hearing loss can be the result of cerumen impaction?

   a. Conductive hearing loss

   b. Sensorineural hearing loss

   c. Noise-induced hearing loss

   d. Mixed hearing loss

12. Upon palpation of the pinna, pain is elicited. The pain worsens when pressure is applied to the tragus. The examiner should suspect:

   a. Acute otitis media

   b. Otitis media with effusion

   c. Otitis externa

   d. Mastoiditis

13. Sensorineural hearing loss is caused by:

   a. Auditory nerve damage

   b. Foreign body in the ear

   c. Impacted cerumen

   d. Perforated tympanic membrane

14. The pediatric health care provider should suspect hearing loss in which of the following children:

    a. A 12-month-old who says only one word
    b. An 18-month-old who says only 20 words
    c. A 6-month-old who does not babble
    d. A 2-year-old whose speech is only 50% intelligible

15. Newborns react to various sounds in all of the following ways *except:*

    a. Demonstrating the acoustic blink reflex
    b. Demonstrating the Moro reflex
    c. Quieting
    d. Demonstrating the Landau reflex

16. Marked erythema of the tympanic membrane in a child can be due to all of the following *except:*

    a. Crying
    b. Fever
    c. Acute otitis media
    d. Heredity

17. Physical examination findings for acute otitis media may include:

    a. Erythematous but mobile tympanic membrane; light reflex present
    b. Erythematous and bulging tympanic membrane; light reflex absent
    c. Dull tympanic membrane with visible air bubbles behind it
    d. Pale, retracted tympanic membrane

18. The health care provider performs a Rinne test on a 15-year-old boy. The teen hears bone conduction longer than air conduction. The provider suspects that the teen has:

    a. Sensorineural hearing loss
    b. Conductive hearing loss
    c. Noise-induced hearing loss
    d. Mixed hearing loss

19. An adolescent complains of tinnitus. All of the following are relevant historical questions to ask *except:*

    a. "What makes the tinnitus better or worse?"
    b. "Have you hit your head recently?"
    c. "Are you on any medications?"
    d. "Are there any close contacts with the same symptoms?"

20. Which of the following drugs are ototoxic?

    a. Gentamycin
    b. Acetaminophen
    c. Prednisolone
    d. Albuterol

SAMPLE DOCUMENTATION: ASSESSMENT OF THE EARS

Patient Name _____ Date of Birth_____ Date_____
Gender_____

I. **Health History**
  A. **Reason for Seeking Health Care** (e.g. routine well-child examination; complaint related to the ear)
    1. Past medical history
      a. Prenatal, birth, neonatal histories (history of aminoglycosides)
      b. Chronic health conditions related to the ear (e.g., acute otitis; otitis media with effusion)
      c. Past hospitalizations (e.g., injuries or infections)
      d. Surgical history (e.g., myringotomy)
      e. Family medical history (e.g., allergies, otitis)
      f. Current medications
      g. Immunization history
      h. Review of systems
    2. History (see *Advanced Pediatric Assessment, Second Edition*, Chapter 14 for age-specific assessment questions)
    3. Developmental history
    4. Social history
  II. **Physical Examination**
  A. **Inspection**
    i. Pinna
    ii. Tympanic membrane (otoscopic examination)
  B. **Palpation**
  C. **Assessment of Hearing Acuity**
  D. **Assessment of Speech**

ASSESSMENT OF THE EARS: WRITE-UP

Use the space provided here to document all subjective and objective findings using the SOAP rubric.

Subjective—(historical information; chief complaint; history of present illness)

_____

_____

Objective—(vital signs, physical examination findings, results of laboratory and other diagnostic tests)

_____

_____

Assessment—(diagnosis [use ICD-10 codes]; other health issues that are identified)

_____

_____

Plan—(treatment, medications, therapies, teaching, referrals, follow-up care)

_____

_____

Assessment of the Eyes

CHAPTER OVERVIEW

This chapter helps to solidify the skills needed to perform an age- and developmentally appropriate examination of the internal and external eye, to assess visual acuity, to recognize deviations from normal, and to accurately record assessment findings.

Expected Learning Outcomes

After reading Chiocca, *Advanced Pediatric Assessment, Second Edition,* Chapter 15, the learner will be able to:

1. Obtain a thorough and accurate pediatric ocular history
2. Examine the external and internal eye and distinguish normal and abnormal findings
3. Identify normal and abnormal findings upon ophthalmoscopic examination
4. Analyze historical and physical assessment findings related to the eye and use these data to make accurate assessments and diagnoses
5. Accurately record history and physical assessment findings related to assessment of the eye

Essential Terminology

Accommodation—a reflex that allows the eye to focus on near objects

Anisocoria—asymmetry of pupil size

Blepharitis—inflammation of the eyelash follicles, causing inflammation of eyelid

Bony orbit—an opening in the skull that surrounds and protects the eyeball

Bruckner test—simultaneous assessment of the red reflex in both pupils

Cataract—opacity of the lens of the eye; can be congenital, caused by prenatal maternal infections, or a genetic or hereditary conditions

Chalazion—painless swelling of the margin of the upper eyelid caused by blockage of the meibomian gland, causing inflammation and erythema

Conjunctiva—a thin, transparent mucous membrane that lines the surface of the inner eyelids and anterior surface of the sclera

Conjunctivitis—inflammation or infection of the conjunctiva

Ectropion—an outward turning of the lower eyelid; can lead to conjunctivitis

Entropion—inversion of the eyelid; a normal finding in Asian children

Exopthalmos—abnormal protrusion of the eye globe

Extraocular muscles—six voluntary muscles that control movement of the eye in the six cardinal fields of gaze and are innervated by cranial nerves III, IV, and VI

Fovea centralis—a pinpoint depression within the macula; the area of the retina with the greatest visual acuity

Glaucoma—an eye condition that raises intraocular pressure

Hordeolum—infection of the sebaceous glands at the base of the eyelash

Inner canthus—the points at which the upper and lower eyelids meet at the left and right sides of each eye

Iris—the colored portion of the eye

Macula—the avascular portion of the ocular fundus located temporal to the optic disc; it is slightly darker than the rest of the fundus and is very sensitive to light

Miosis—pupillary constriction

Nystagmus—involuntary, rapid, lateral eye movements

Optic disc—the location where the optic nerve enters the eye

Optic foramen—an opening through which the optic nerve, ophthalmic artery, and ophthalmic vein from each eye pass to the brain

Palpebral fissure—the longitudinal opening between the upper and lower eyelids

Papilledema—swelling of the optic disc; evident when the disc margins are blurry or obliterated and the physiologic cup cannot be seen; caused by increased intracranial pressure

Ptosis—drooping of the upper eyelid

Puncta—small openings in the inner canthus that permit the drainage of tears

Pupil—center part of the iris; sphincter and dilator muscles allow the pupil to increase (dilate) and decrease (constrict) in size to control the amount of light entering the eye

Red reflex—a reflection of the retinal background elicited when an ophthalmoscope light is shined on the pupil

Retina—the light-sensitive, innermost layer of the eye

Retinopathy of prematurity—poor vision or blindness caused by perinatal hypoxia

Sclera—the white part of the eye; an opaque, firm, fibrous tissue that coats the outer eye and is visible just beneath the conjunctiva

Strabismus—ocular misalignment

Label the anatomic structures indicated on these illustrations.

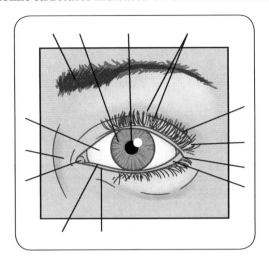

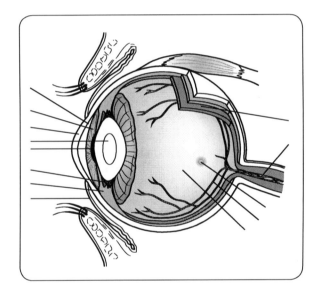

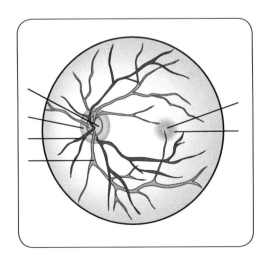

CRITICAL THINKING EXERCISES

Short-Answer Critical Thinking Exercises

1. Describe and discuss the developmental variations and age-related variability in the eye and vision.
2. Fill in the box with the age- and developmentally relevant well-child eye and vision examination.

AGE	ASSESSMENTS
Neonate	
6 months to 3 years	
3 to 5 years	
6 years and older	

3. At what age is an asymmetrical corneal light reflex no longer within normal limits?
4. What is the possible consequence of untreated strabismus?
5. What are some subjective and objective signs that a child may have a vision abnormality?
6. State the normal and abnormal findings of the fundoscopic exam. At what age should the examiner begin the fundoscopic exam as part of the well-child visit?
7. What are some aspects of the infant's or child's past medical history that may affect his or her vision?
8. Name some common ocular complaints in children.
9. What are the six cardinal fields of gaze? Discuss how these findings relates to assessment of the eye.
10. Describe and explain the pupillary light reflex. What is the direct and consensual light reflex?

Critical Thinking Case Study Exercises

Exercise 1

For each age group listed here, identify the eye and vision assessments that should be performed at each health maintenance visit:

1. 0 to 6 months
2. 6 to 12 months
3. 1 to 2 years
4. 2 to 5 years
5. 5 to 10 years
6. 10 and older

Exercise 2

Truman is an 8-year-old boy whose parents bring him to the urgent care center with complaints of severe right eyelid swelling and fever for 2 days. His parents say his symptoms have worsened, and when he woke up this morning, he had blurred vision.

1. What other information should the health care provider gather about the history of present illness (HPI)?
2. What other objective assessments are necessary to obtain on Truman?
3. What should the physical examination focus on?
4. What is your differential diagnosis?

Exercise 3

Mary, aged 10 years, is in the office for her annual physical, accompanied by her mother and two younger siblings. When the mother is asked if she has any concerns, she says yes; Mary rubs her eyes often and when she does, her eyelids appear swollen and puffy, the "whites of her eyes get all red, and clear stuff comes out that looks like tears."

1. Once the physical is completed and you focus on Mary's eye complaint, what other questions should you ask Mary and her mother about her eye complaint?
2. Is there anything in Mary's past medical history that you would want to know that would help you make a diagnosis?
3. Is there anything in Mary's family history that you would want to know that would help you make a diagnosis?
4. Is there anything you should ask about or observe in Mary's siblings that is relevant?

Exercise 4

Jackson is a 4-year-old boy who was playing in the sandbox about an hour ago. He is now complaining of moderate to severe eye pain and is crying.

1. What historical data should be gathered?
2. What should the physical assessment include?
3. Should any specific testing be done?
4. What diagnosis do you suspect?

REVIEW QUESTIONS

1. Objective measurements of visual acuity begin at age:

   a. 6 months
   b. 1 year
   c. 2 years
   d. 3 years

2. At the 9-month visit, the eye exam is done, and the following findings are documented. Which of the findings listed below is *not* within normal limits?

   a. Bilateral red reflex present
   b. Asymmetrical corneal lite reflex (Hirschberg test)
   c. Positive blink reflex
   d. Demonstrated binocular fix and follow

3. A 2-year-old has 20/50 vision. The provider's assessment of this is:

   a. It is within normal limits for the child's age
   b. The child needs a referral to an ophthalmologist
   c. The child has decreased binocular vision
   d. The child may have problems with accommodation and convergence

4. The mother of a 6-year-old boy brings the child to the clinic stating that he woke up that morning with "his eye glued shut" with sticky, yellow drainage. She says that she used a warm, wet washcloth to "unglue" his eye. Upon questioning, she states that she received a note from the school nurse stating that two children in her son's class had "pink-eye." The provider inspects the affected eye, and expects the conjunctiva to appear:

   a. Clear, smooth, moist, and whitish
   b. Cloudy with a bluish tinge
   c. Watery with a yellowish tinge
   d. Injected and inflamed, with a small amount of clear to pale yellow drainage

5. The area of the ocular fundus that is slightly darker than the rest of the fundus and is very sensitive to light is the:

   a. Optic disc
   b. Macula
   c. Physiologic cup
   d. Oculus

6. Which of the following may indicate a problem with a school-aged child's vision?

   a. Uses finger to maintain place when reading
   b. Prefers reading to watching television
   c. Can see clearly and comfortably at 10 to 13 inches
   d. Is aware of things located to the side while looking straight ahead

7. The pediatric health care provider would need to refer an infant with continuous esotropia at age:

   a. 2 months
   b. 4 months
   c. 6 months
   d. 9 months

8. The ophthalmoscopic examination should be part of the routine assessment beginning at age:

   a. 6 months
   b. 1 year
   c. 3 years
   d. 5 years

9. The "tumbling E" chart is used to measure visual acuity in what age group?

   a. 18 months to 2 years
   b. 1 to 2 years
   c. 2 to 3 years
   d. 3 to 5 years

10. During the physical examination portion of the well-child visit for an 18-month-old, the provider notes leukocoria. This finding:

    a. Is normal and requires no action
    b. Is normal if there is a family history of leukocoria
    c. Is equivocal and the child should be re-examined in 6 months
    d. Requires an immediate referral to a pediatric ophthalmologist

11. Thad is a 6-year-old boy who has had only episodic health care since birth. He presents to the clinic for a kindergarten physical. One physical finding is marked, intermittent esotropia of the left eye. You recommend an immediate referral to a pediatric ophthalmologist. Thad's mother is skeptical, stating that "he has always had a lazy eye and no one said anything before. Why should he get checked now?" You respond by saying that:

    a. If it is inconvenient for you to get to the ophthalmologist, it can wait
    b. It is important that Thad get checked before his other eye is affected
    c. Thad must see an ophthalmologist immediately to be evaluated and treated to prevent neurologic blindness in his left eye
    d. If Thad has had a "lazy eye" for this long and seems fine, he does not need an ophthalmology referral

12. A 14-year-old child is seen in the school-based clinic because of a swollen, painless area on the upper eyelid. This finding is most likely:

    a. Chalazion
    b. Keratitis
    c. Cellulitis
    d. Uveitis

13. Upon examination of the eye, a 6-month-old has a white instead of red reflex in the left eye. This may be indicative of:

    a. Papilledema
    b. Diplopia
    c. Strabismus
    d. Retinoblastoma

14. The cover/uncover test is used for detecting:

    a. Nystagmus
    b. Cataracts
    c. Strabismus
    d. Astigmatism

15. Nystagmus can be a normal finding in which age group?

    a. Neonate
    b. Infant
    c. Toddler
    d. Adolescent

16. The absence of the red reflex can indicate:

    a. Retinoblastoma
    b. Glaucoma
    c. Astigmatism
    d. Amblyopia

17. A school nurse practitioner has completed vision screening for a group of preschoolers. All children were screened with the HOTV chart. Which of the following children should be referred for further testing?

    a. A 3-year-old who screened 20/30 in the left eye; 20/20 in the right eye
    b. A 3-year-old who screened 20/30 in the left eye; 20/30 in the right eye
    c. A 4-year-old who screened 20/40 in the left eye; 20/30 in the right eye
    d. A 4-year-old who screened 20/30 in the left eye; 20/30 in the right eye

18. The simultaneous constriction of the pupil in the contralateral eye when the other pupil is exposed to bright light is:

    a. Accommodation
    b. Consensual light reflex
    c. Bruckner test
    d. Hirschberg test

19. Absence of the blink reflex suggests:

    a. Decreased peripheral vision
    b. Impaired accommodation
    c. Impaired light perception
    d. Impaired binocular vision

20. To evaluate peripheral vision in a young child, which of the following tests is done?

    a. Confrontation test
    b. Hirschberg test
    c. HOTV test
    d. Ishihara's test

SAMPLE DOCUMENTATION: ASSESSMENT OF THE EYES

Patient Name _____ Date of Birth_____ Date_____
Gender_____

I. **Health History**
   A. **Reason for Seeking Health Care** (e.g., routine well-child examination; eye infection or injury)
   1. Past medical history
      a. Prenatal, birth, neonatal histories
      b. Chronic health conditions related to the eye
      c. Past hospitalizations (e.g., eye injuries or infections)
      d. Surgical history (e.g., strabismus, cataracts, or an injury to the eye)
      e. Family medical history (e.g., genetic or metabolic disorders)
      f. Current medications
      g. Immunization history
      h. Review of systems
   2. Ocular history (see *Advanced Pediatric Assessment, Second Edition*, Chapter 15, for age-specific assessment questions)
   3. Developmental history
   4. Social history

II. **Physical Examination**
   A. **Inspection of Facies, Eye Placement**
   B. **Inspection of External Eye Structures**
   C. **Inspection of Anterior Globe (Eyeball) Structures**
   D. **Assessment of Extraocular Muscle Function**
   1. Corneal light reflex (the Hirschberg Test)
   2. Cross-cover test
   3. Six cardinal fields of gaze
   4. Testing of convergence
   E. **Assessment of Visual Acuity**
   F. **Assessment of Color Vision**
   G. **Assessment of Visual Fields**
   H. **Inspection of Ocular Fundus; Ophthalmoscopic Exam**
   I. **Palpation of External Eye Structures**

ASSESSMENT OF THE EYES: WRITE-UP

Use the space provided here to document all subjective and objective findings using the SOAP rubric.

Subjective—(historical information; chief complaint; history of present illness)

_____

_____

Objective—(vital signs, physical examination findings, results of laboratory and other diagnostic tests)

_____

_____

Assessment—(diagnosis [use ICD-10 codes]; other health issues that are identified)

_____

_____

Plan—(treatment, medications, therapies, teaching, referrals, follow-up care)

_____

_____

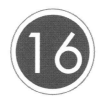

Assessment of the Face, Nose, and Oral Cavity

CHAPTER OVERVIEW

This chapter helps the pediatric health care provider to conduct an age- and developmentally appropriate examination of the face, nose, and oral cavity; to recognize deviations from normal; and to accurately record assessment findings.

Expected Learning Outcomes

After reading Chiocca, *Advanced Pediatric Assessment, Second Edition,* Chapter 16, the learner will be able to:

1. Obtain a thorough and accurate history related to the face, nose, and oral cavity in the pediatric patient
2. Accurately conduct an age- and developmentally appropriate physical examination of the face, nose, and oral cavity in the pediatric patient and distinguish normal and abnormal findings
3. Analyze historical and physical assessment findings related to the face, nose, and oral cavity and use these data to make accurate assessments and diagnoses
4. Accurately record history and physical assessment findings related to assessment of the face, nose, and oral cavity

Essential Terminology

Buccal mucosa—the tissue lining the inside of the cheeks

Candidiasis—adherent white plaques on the buccal mucosa due to a fungal infection

Caries—tooth decay

"Cobblestoning"—streaks of lymphoid tissue on the posterior pharynx, which have the appearance of cobblestones; often seen with allergic rhinitis

Deciduous teeth—the first set of teeth; begin to erupt at approximately age 6 months and exfoliate between 6 and 12 years of age

Epistaxis—nosebleed

Hard palate—the anterior two thirds of the palate; made of bone

Hypopharynx—the area of the pharynx that extends from the level of the hyoid bone to the inferior border of the cricoid cartilage

Koplik's spots—tiny bluish-white dots surrounded by red halos on the buccal mucosa; considered pathognomonic for the onset of measles

Lingual frenulum—mucosal tissue that attaches the tongue to the floor of the mouth

Nasal vestibule—the internal nose

Nasopharynx—the superior portion of the pharynx (throat); continuous with the oropharynx

Oropharynx—the portion of the pharynx between the soft palate and the upper portion of the epiglottis

Palate—the structure that separates the nasal and oral cavities and forms the roof of the mouth

Palatine tonsils—lymphoid tissue, located on either side of the oropharynx, just behind the arches of the soft palate

Paranasal sinuses—air pockets on either side of the nasal cavity

Pharyngeal tonsils (adenoids)—lymph tissue located on the superior posterior wall of the nasopharynx

Pharynx—the entry to the trachea and esophagus; the throat

Philtrum—a midline, vertical groove between the base of the nose and upper lip

Soft palate—the posterior third of the palate; it is composed of muscle and is part of the lateral pharyngeal wall

Turbinates—bony projections located in the lateral wall of each nasal cavity; nasal turbinates are highly vascular and lined with cilia and mucous membranes; they serve to increase surface area to warm and humidify inhaled air

Uvula—the vertical muscular structure that hangs from the middle of the soft palate

Label the anatomic structures indicated on these illustrations.

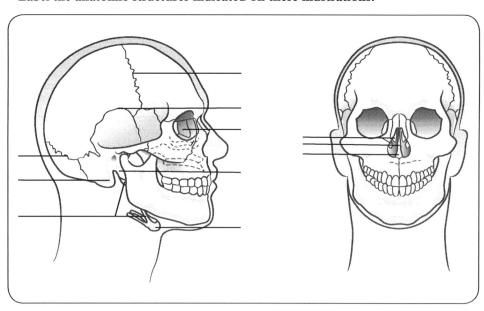

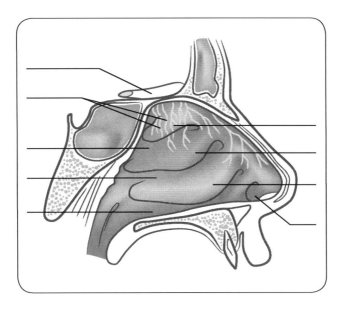

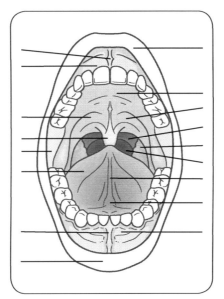

CRITICAL THINKING EXERCISES

Short-Answer Critical Thinking Exercises

1. Discuss the clinical implications of the young infant being an obligate nose breather.
2. Discuss neonatal assessment of the face, nose, and oral cavity and the foci of each.
3. How do the prenatal, perinatal, and neonatal histories affect the assessment of the face, nose, and mouth in infants and children?
4. What vaccine-preventable illnesses can cause medical conditions that affect the face, nose, sinuses, or oral cavity?

5. Discuss aspects of the past medical history that are relevant to the face, nose, and oral cavity.
6. Discuss aspects of the past surgical history that are relevant to the face, nose, and oral cavity.
7. What aspects of the social history are relevant to the face, nose, and oral cavity?
8. Discuss the elements of the oral and dental history in the pediatric patient.
9. Discuss the elements of the pediatric oral health risk assessment.
10. Discuss some physical examination techniques that can be helpful when examining the nose and mouth in infants and young children.
11. List the elements of the pediatric physical assessment of the face, nose, and oral cavity.

Critical Thinking Case Study Exercises

Exercise 1

Jenna is a 4-year-old girl whose mother brings her to the clinic, stating that she has a cold. Jenna has been sneezing, and her mother states that she coughs more at night when she goes to bed. Physical examination reveals boggy, pale nasal mucosa with clear nasal drainage.

1. What would you like to know about Jenna's medical history?
2. Would you ask any other questions with respect to her history of present illness?
3. What specific physical assessments would you make?
4. What diagnosis do you suspect?

Exercise 2

A 10-year-old child presents with a 1-day history of erythematous, 3+ tonsils, and petechiae on the soft palate. Yellowish-white exudate is seen on an erythematous posterior pharynx.

1. What other historical data are important to know?
2. What objective data are important to know?
3. What should the physical examination focus on?
4. Should any diagnostic testing be done?
5. What condition do you suspect?

Exercise 3

A 5-day-old infant girl has white patches on the buccal mucosa. The infant just finished feeding 4 ounces of formula.

1. What other historical data are important to know?
2. What objective data are important to know?
3. What further assessments should be made on the white patches in the infant's mouth?
4. Should any other physical assessments be made?
5. What condition do you suspect?

Exercise 4

Matthew is an 18-month-old toddler who presents for his well-child health maintenance examination. While obtaining the history, the provider notes that Matthew has not been weaned from the bottle, and drinks four to six bottles of apple juice per day. Matthew's basal metabolic index falls on the 97th percentile on the growth charts.

1. List the questions that you would ask Matthew's mother regarding his oral and dental history.
2. Would you conduct an oral health risk assessment?
3. What specific assessments would you conduct when you examine Matthew's teeth?

REVIEW QUESTIONS

1. Assessment of the face begins with:

   a. Inspection of the skin for color, lesions, and signs of trauma or edema
   b. Inspection of the facies, noting the size, shape, symmetry, and spacing of facial features
   c. Palpation of the face for swelling or pain
   d. Bimanual palpation of the mandible and maxilla

2. A 1-month-old infant is brought to the clinic for a well-child visit. On examination of the mouth white, cottage cheese–like patches on the inner aspect of the buccal mucosa are noted. This is likely cause by:

   a. Herpangina
   b. Oral candidiasis
   c. Immunodeficiency
   d. Prolonged bottle feeding

3. Nasal turbinates that are edematous and erythematous are likely indicative of:

   a. Upper respiratory infection
   b. Allergic rhinitis
   c. Sinusitis
   d. Foreign body

4. Tonsils that are unequal in size can indicate the presence of a(n):

   a. Peritonsillar abscess
   b. Streptococcal pharyngitis
   c. Epiglottitis
   d. Infectious mononucleosis

5. When examining a child, the examiner notes that the child has an absent philtrum and depressed nasal bridge. The examiner suspects:

   a. Allergic rhinitis
   b. Fetal alcohol syndrome

    c. Pierre Robin sequence

    d. Marfan syndrome

6. Inspection of the internal nose begins by:

    a. Inspecting the inferior and middle nasal turbinates

    b. Inspecting the nares for patency

    c. Inspecting the nares for drainage

    d. Inspecting the nasal septum for alignment

7. An 18-month-old toddler has black and brown spots on his central maxillary and mandibular incisors. You suspect:

    a. Oral injury

    b. Gingivitis

    c. Early childhood caries

    d. Xerostomia

8. Which of the following is not considered a risk factor for tooth decay in children?

    a. Propping the bottle for feedings

    b. High consumption of fruit

    c. High consumption of sweetened drinks

    d. The use of a no-spill sippy cup

9. Infants are obligate nose breathers until age:

    a. 1 month

    b. 2 months

    c. 3 months

    d. 4 months

10. The first deciduous teeth that erupt are typically the:

    a. Central mandibular incisors

    b. Central maxillary incisors

    c. Maxillary lateral incisors

    d. Mandibular lateral incisors

11. Tonsils that are enlarged and meet halfway between tonsillar pillars and uvula would be graded:

    a. 1+

    b. 2+

    c. 3+

    d. 4+

12. A nasal quality to a child's speech may indicate:

    a. Submucosal cleft palate

    b. Dental caries

    c. Transitional dentition

    d. Peritonsillar abscess

13. Joseph, 4 years old, has dark, bluish circles under the eyes, a lateral crease on his nose, and is frequently sniffing during the health care encounter. Which of the following conditions do you suspect?

    a. Nasopharyngitis

    b. Sinusitis

    c. Allergic rhinitis

    d. Nasal foreign body

14. Mixed dentition can place a child at risk for:

    a. Plaque accumulation

    b. Dental fractures

    c. Tooth avulsions

    d. Otitis media

15. Erythematous macules that evolve into vesicles that ulcerate are likely:

    a. Streptococcal pharyngitis

    b. Herpangina

    c. Retropharyngeal abscess

    d. Cervical adenitis

16. Tooth decalcification, erosion, and decay in an underweight adolescent girl raises suspicion for:

    a. Anorexia nervosa

    b. Bulimia nervosa

    c. Use of chewing tobacco

    d. Chronic alcohol use

17. Finger or thumb sucking in a child can affect dental arch development, resulting in malocclusion after approximately what age?

    a. 1 year

    b. 3 years

    c. 5 years

    d. 7 years

18. Unilateral rhinorrhea is likely caused by:

    a. Nasopharyngitis

    b. Foreign body in the nose

    c. Allergic rhinitis

    d. Sinusitis

19. Gum recession and leukoplakia in a male adolescent raise suspicion for the use of:

    a. Chewing tobacco
    b. Methamphetamine use
    c. Inhaled cocaine use
    d. Marijuana use

20. In a medical record, the tonsils are graded as 4+. When the mouth of this child is examined, the tonsils would be:

    a. Visible
    b. Halfway between the tonsillar pillars and uvula
    c. Touching the uvula
    d. Touching at the midline

SAMPLE DOCUMENTATION: ASSESSMENT OF THE FACE, NOSE, AND ORAL CAVITY

Patient Name _____ Date of Birth_____ Date_____
Gender_____

I. **Health History**
   A. **Reason for Seeking Health Care** (e.g. routine well-child examination; complaint related to the face, nose, and oral cavity)
      1. Past medical history
         a. Prenatal, birth, neonatal histories
         b. Chronic health conditions
         c. Past hospitalizations
         d. Injuries
         e. Surgical history
         f. Family medical history
         g. Current medications
         h. Allergy history
         i. Immunization history
         j. Dental history
         k. Review of systems
      2. Developmental history
      3. Social history
      4. Oral health risk assessment

II. **Physical Examination**
   A. **Face**
      1. Inspection
      2. Palpation
      3. Percussion (sinuses)
   B. **Nose**
      1. Inspection
      2. Palpation

    C. Oral Cavity
        1. Inspection
        2. Palpation

ASSESSMENT OF THE FACE, NOSE, AND ORAL CAVITY: WRITE-UP

Use the space provided here to document all subjective and objective findings using the SOAP rubric.

Subjective—(historical information; chief complaint; history of present illness)

_____

_____

Objective—(vital signs, physical examination findings, results of laboratory and other diagnostic tests)

_____

_____

Assessment—(diagnosis [use ICD-10 codes]; other health issues that are identified)

_____

_____

Plan—(treatment, medications, therapies, teaching, referrals, follow-up care)

_____

_____

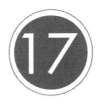

Assessment of the Thorax, Lungs, and Regional Lymphatics

CHAPTER OVERVIEW

Respiratory infections and disorders are very common in children. Therefore, the pediatric health care provider must be able to obtain a complete respiratory history and perform a thorough respiratory physical examination. Important skills include being adept in inspection, auscultation palpation, and percussion in order to formulate accurate differential diagnoses. This chapter also reviews developmental approaches to the respiratory physical assessment that are important, especially for younger children.

Expected Learning Outcomes

After reading Chiocca, *Advanced Pediatric Assessment, Second Edition,* Chapter 17, the learner will be able to:

1. Demonstrate the ability to obtain an accurate and thorough respiratory health history for all pediatric age groups
2. Perform an accurate and thorough physical examination of the respiratory system for all pediatric age groups
3. Identify and differentiate normal and abnormal breath sounds in infants and children
4. Recognize signs of respiratory distress in infants, children, and adolescents
5. Demonstrate the ability to record all health assessment findings accurately and completely

Essential Terminology

Adventitious—"extra" breath sounds; for example, wheezes

Alveoli—small, balloon-like structures in the lung where gas exchange takes place

Apnea—cessation of respiration

Asthma—a chronic, inflammatory respiratory disorder characterized by airway inflammation, airflow obstruction, and airway hyperresponsiveness

Atelectasis—the condition in which alveoli are collapsed; results in diminished or absent gas exchange

Barrel chest—a rounded, barrel shape of the chest due to chronic hyperinflation

Bradypnea—abnormally slow respiratory rate; in children the normal respiratory rate is age dependent, thus definition of bradypnea will vary

Bronchial—a normal breath sound heard over the trachea and thorax; short during inspiration, long during expiration, and high in pitch

Bronchiole—a smaller division of the bronchus; a thin-walled, cylindrical structure that further divides into alveoli

Bronchiolitis—lower respiratory tract inflammation, edema, and mucous production, usually caused by a viral infection; occurs mainly in children from birth to age 2 years

Bronchophony—an assessment of the spoken voice through the stethoscope; the child is asked to say "99"; with normal lung tissue, voice sounds heard through the stethoscope are muffled; with lung consolidation, the voice sounds are clear

Bronchovesicular—a normal breath sound heard over the major bronchi; heard posteriorly between the scapulae and anteriorly around the upper sternum; of equal duration during inspiration and expiration, and moderate in pitch

Central cyanosis—cyanosis along the midline

Cilia—fine, sweeping, hair-like projections that line the respiratory tract; their function is to move fluids and particles up and out

Clubbing—a condition in which the angle of the fingernails and nail beds becomes convex over time; caused by chronic hypoxia

Consolidation—an area of lung tissue filled with fluid or exudate

Crackles—high-pitched, soft, crackling (fine crackles) or low-pitched, gurgling (coarse crackles) lung sounds, may be localized or diffuse; heard on inspiration; clear with cough

Crepitus—crackling or popping sensation upon palpation of the chest

Cyanosis—bluish skin color caused by hypoxemia

Dead space—areas of the respiratory tract in which gas exchange does not take place; for example, the trachea and bronchi

Diaphragmatic breathing—respirations in which the abdomen rises with inspiration

Dyspnea—difficulty breathing

Egophony—a sound produced upon auscultation when assessing for lung consolidation; the child is asked to say "ee"; with normal lung findings, the sound is muffled; with lung consolidation, the sound produced sounds like "ay"

Excursion—a lung palpation technique to assess for symmetrical chest expansion

Fremitus—the presence of palpable chest vibrations when a child speaks or an infant cries

Grunting—the sound produced when the glottis closes during expiration; most often occurs in neonates and young infants; accompanies prolonged expiration and is often a sign of carbon dioxide retention; grunting is a sign of respiratory distress and is never within normal limits

Hyperventilation—rapid, deep breathing

Hypoxemia—decreased level of oxygen in the blood

Intercostal—between the ribs

Kussmaul's breathing—deep and labored breathing caused by metabolic acidosis

Mottling—patchy bluish-purple areas of the skin; may be caused by cool ambient room temperatures, vasoconstriction, or hypoxemia; skin may also be cool to touch with delayed capillary refill depending on etiology of mottling; may be within normal limits in the immediate neonatal period

Orthopnea—difficulty breathing while lying flat that is relieved by sitting in an upright position

Paradoxical breathing—respirations in which the diaphragm falls rather than rises during inspiration

Pectus carinatum—a congenital protuberant chest wall deformity

Pectus excavatum—a congenital depression of the chest wall

Percussion—striking the chest wall with sharp but gentle finger blows to assess and locate air, fluid, or masses in the lung; also done to locate organ boundaries

Periodic breathing—periods of apnea; up to 20 seconds is within normal limits for neonates

Peripheral cyanosis—cyanosis seen on the hands, feet, or around the mouth

Pleural friction rub—a low-pitched, grating, or creaking sound; loudest on inspiration; occurs when inflamed pleura rub together

Posttussive—after coughing

Retractions—the use of accessory chest muscles for breathing

Rhonchi—a low-pitched, snore-like, adventitious lung sound caused by airway narrowing and blockage of secretions; often improves after coughing or secretion removal

Stridor—a loud, coarse, high-pitched sound caused by upper airway narrowing or inflammation

Subcostal—below the ribs

Substernal—below the sternum

Supraclavicular—above the clavicle(s)

Suprasternal—above the sternum

Tachypnea—abnormally rapid respiratory rate; in children the normal respiratory rate is age dependent, thus definition of tachypnea will vary

Vesicular—a soft, low-pitched, normal breath sound heard in peripheral lung fields

Wheezes—high-pitched whistling, musical, or squeaky breath sounds caused by airway narrowing

Whispered pectoriloquy—a sound produced upon auscultation when assessing for lung consolidation; the child is asked to whisper "99" several times while the examiner auscultates all lung fields; increased loudness is auscultated over consolidated lung tissue; a faint sound is heard over normal lung tissue

Xiphoid process—a small, cartilaginous tip at the lower part of the sternum

CRITICAL THINKING EXERCISES

Short-Answer Critical Thinking Exercises

1. What are some anatomic and physiologic differences in the respiratory system of infants and children compared with that of adults? How do some of these differences affect respiratory function in the infant or child?
2. What are the essential questions to ask when obtaining a respiratory health history for an infant? Do the questions change when a child is older? Why or why not? Which questions change or stay the same?
3. When obtaining the review of systems, which body systems are important to include when assessing the respiratory system in children?
4. What are some vaccine-preventable illnesses that affect the respiratory system in children?
5. Why is it important to know a child's allergy history as part of the respiratory assessment?
6. Why is the social history an important part of the respiratory assessment?
7. Explicate how vital signs reflect the infant or child's respiratory status and vice versa.
8. Name the parts of the respiratory physical exam that are included during inspection.
9. Explain retractions, their cause, and where on the chest they can be assessed. Discuss whether the location or severity of the retractions is related to the diagnosis.
10. What does the tripod position indicate? What are some pediatric respiratory conditions that may cause a child to assume the tripod position?
11. Explain, step by step, the sequence of chest auscultation in infants and children.
12. Name and describe each of the three normal breath sounds.
13. Name and describe abnormal and adventitious breath sounds in infants and children, and give an example of an associated condition for each.
14. When assessing a quiet infant or toddler, why should the provider auscultate the chest first before any other assessment?
15. Why is chest palpation conducted as part of the respiratory assessment in children? What is assessed?

16. Why is chest percussion conducted as part of the respiratory assessment in children? What are the various percussion notes that may be elicited and the meaning of each?
17. Discuss some signs of chronic respiratory disease in children and what these signs indicate.
18. Why are respiratory diagnoses so common in infants and young children?

Critical Thinking Case Study Exercises

Exercise 1

Cooper is a 15-month-old toddler in the clinic for his health supervision visit. His past medical history includes three past hospital admissions for wheezing, and both parents smoke in the home. While gathering the historical data, the health care provider thinks she may have heard audible wheezes, but Copper's nares are both filled with crusted mucous and he is breathing through his nose. When it is time to examine him, Cooper cries, clings to his mother, arches, and becomes very uncooperative.

1. In what order should Copper's physical examination be conducted?
2. Should Cooper be examined on his mother's lap or on the exam table?
3. What are some techniques that can be used to obtain the most accurate auscultation findings possible?
4. Given the scenario in this exercise, why is it especially important to obtain the most accurate auscultation findings possible on Cooper?

Exercise 2

Timothy is an 8-month-old European American infant. He is brought to the emergency room by his teenage mother. She states that Timothy is unable to take his bottle because he cannot breathe out of his nose. She says he has been crying "his hungry cry," but every time she tries to feed him, he spits the bottle out and acts like he can't breathe. General inspection of Timothy reveals an alert, well-nourished infant. He is pink and in no acute respiratory distress. Both nares have copious amounts of thick, dried, green nasal discharge.

1. What other historical questions should be asked of Timothy's mother?
2. What priority assessment(s) should be conducted next?
3. Should any intervention be conducted before proceeding with the physical examination?
4. In what order should the objective data be collected?
5. Is there anything else in the general survey that is important to assess?
6. What teaching should Timothy's mother receive?

Exercise 3

Nora is a 4-year-old girl who presents to the clinic with her mother. Her mother states that Nora has been coughing at night for approximately a month. Nora is smiling, happy, and friendly. The examiner bends over to admire Nora's artwork, and hears audible wheezing. The examiner then looks at the chart and notes that all vital signs are within normal limits.

1. What are the important elements to include in the history of present illness for Nora?
2. What are the important elements to include in Nora's past medical history?
3. Is Nora's family medical history relevant in this particular instance? Why or why not?
4. Discuss why it is important to gather information on Nora's medication, hospitalization, immunization, and allergy history. How does this information relate to the differential diagnoses?
5. What questions regarding the social history are important to ask?
6. What should Nora's physical examination focus on?
7. Describe what should be included in Nora's respiratory assessment.
8. What particular physical assessments should be made that may be relevant to Nora's diagnosis?

Exercise 4

Juan Carlos is a 4-year-old Honduran boy who is brought by his grandmother to the emergency room because of a severe sore throat and fever. He is dyspneic, drooling, and looks frightened. Through an interpreter, the provider asks Juan Carlos's grandmother some questions. The answers reveal that Juan Carlos has no known allergies, has not ingested anything, is not on any medication, and has no chronic illnesses. Juan Carlos has not received any immunizations. Vital signs are temperature 103.2°F (39.5°C); pulse 128 bpm; respiratory rate 32 and labored; blood pressure 102/66. Oxygen saturation is 92%.

1. What assessment should come next? What assessment should *not* be made?
2. Juan Carlos has no cough. Is this respiratory assessment significant? Why or why not?
3. Juan Carlos's voice sounds muffled when he tries to speak. Is this respiratory assessment significant? Why or why not?
4. Is the fact that Juan Carlos is drooling an important assessment? Why or why not?
5. Juan Carlos is now sitting upright, mouth open, jaw thrust forward, with his tongue hanging out. What is this position called? What causes a patient to assume this position? What should be done next for Juan Carlos?

Refer to Figures 17.10 and Figure 17.12 in the textbook. Fill in the blank circles for each illustration that follows with a number to illustrate the correct sequence for auscultation of the lungs.

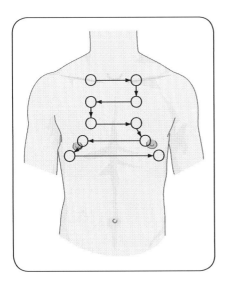 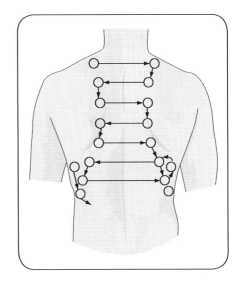

REVIEW QUESTIONS

1. Localization of breath sounds in neonates and infants is often difficult due to:

   a. Large thoracic size
   b. Poor transmission of breath sounds
   c. Small size of nasal passages
   d. Thin chest wall

2. Exacerbation of cough with exercise suggests:

   a. Allergic rhinitis
   b. Asthma
   c. Gastroesophageal reflux disease
   d. Sinusitis

3. A child comes to the clinic with a history of a chronic cough. His history is positive for contact with an adult with a chronic cough. This suggests the possibility of:

   a. Pertussis
   b. Bronchitis
   c. Foreign body in the nose
   d. Acute rhinovirus

4. Auscultation of crackles (rales) is associated with all of the following respiratory conditions *except*:

   a. Pneumonia
   b. Bronchiolitis
   c. Pneumothorax
   d. Atelectasis

5. Percussion of a child's or an adolescent's chest is done to:

   a. Locate air, fluid, or masses
   b. Assess pain
   c. Evaluate respiratory excursion
   d. Assess tactile fremitus

6. Stridor is associated with which of the following respiratory conditions in children?

   a. Epiglottitis
   b. Pertussis
   c. Asthma
   d. Laryngotracheobronchitis

7. The normal respiratory rate of a 2-year-old child is:

   a. 12 to 20 breaths/minute
   b. 14 to 22 breaths/minute
   c. 20 to 30 breaths/minute
   d. 30 to 45 breaths/minute

8. All of the following findings may be indicative of impending respiratory failure in an infant or child *except*:

   a. Expiratory grunting
   b. Cough
   c. Drooling
   d. Assuming the tripod position

9. Finger clubbing is associated with:

   a. Atopy
   b. Respiratory infection
   c. Respiratory distress
   d. Chronic hypoxia

10. When auscultating a child's lungs, a high-pitched, musical sound is heard on expiration. This breath sound is:

    a. Crackles
    b. Wheezing
    c. Stridor
    d. Rhonchi

11. Suprasternal retractions are most likely to be seen with:

    a. Epiglottitis
    b. Asthma
    c. Pneumonia
    d. Tuberculosis

12. In children from birth to age 2 years, respiratory syncytial virus (RSV) can cause:

   a. Asthma
   b. Bronchiolitis
   c. Tracheitis
   d. Croup

13. Which of the following describes the characteristics of the cough that occurs with pertussis?

   a. High-pitched; occurs on inspiration; makes a whooping sound
   b. High-pitched; occurs on inspiration; makes a barking sound
   c. Low-pitched, frequent, dry cough
   d. Low-pitched, frequent, productive cough

14. Signs of chronic respiratory disease in a child may include:

   a. Retractions
   b. Nasal flaring
   c. Barrel-shaped chest
   d. Assuming the tripod position

15. A 15-year-old boy complains of chest and back pain and decreased stamina when wall-climbing in gym class. After exercise, he experiences shortness of breath. His medical history is positive for gastroesophageal reflux and asthma, and pulmonary function testing revealed both restrictive and obstructive disease. Upon inspection, the examiner notes a significant depression of the chest wall in the sternal region. No other physical findings are observed. This chest wall deformity is likely:

   a. Scoliosis
   b. Marfan syndrome
   c. Pectus carinatum
   d. Pectus excavatum

16. Physical examination techniques that may assist in the auscultation of a child's lungs include all of the following *except*:

   a. Placing an infant or toddler on the parent's lap during auscultation
   b. Allowing the child to listen through the stethoscope at what the provider hears
   c. Using a pediatric stethoscope on all children, despite age or weight
   d. Ensuring a quiet atmosphere in order to yield the most accurate findings

17. All of the following describe the correct routine when auscultating the lungs of a pediatric patient *except*:

   a. Auscultate for one full respiratory cycle
   b. Auscultate over the young child's clothes or examination gown to maximize the child's cooperation
   c. Auscultate over all lung fields, anteriorly, posteriorly, and laterally
   d. Auscultate the child's lungs systematically, moving side to side

18. Which lymph nodes are palpated during a full assessment of the thorax?

    a. Supraclavicular and axillary
    b. Preauricular and postauricular
    c. Submental and cervical
    d. Cervical and submaxillary

19. Causes of chest pain in children may include all of the following *except*:

    a. Pneumonia
    b. Costochondritis
    c. Pericarditis
    d. Pertussis

20. An 8-year-old child has been diagnosed with pneumonia on the basis of a chest radiograph. The radiology report states that the child has an area of consolidation in the left lower lobe (LLL). When auscultating this child's lungs over the LLL, the respiratory findings most likely to be found upon auscultation are:

    a. Wheezes
    b. Diminished
    c. Crackles
    d. Rhonchi

SAMPLE DOCUMENTATION: ASSESSMENT OF THE RESPIRATORY SYSTEM

Patient Name _____ Date of Birth_____ Date_____
Gender_____

I. **Health History**
   A. **Prenatal History**
      1. Maternal smoking during pregnancy
      2. Maternal alcohol or recreational drug use
         a. Type of drugs used
         b. Frequency of use
      3. Diagnosed genetic illnesses (e.g., cystic fibrosis)
   B. **Perinatal History**
      1. Birth weight and gestational age
      2. Prematurity
      3. Fetal distress/apnea
      4. Hypoxia/asphyxia
      5. Meconium or amniotic fluid aspiration
      6. Cyanosis at birth requiring oxygen
      7. Apgar scores
   C. **Postnatal History**
      1. Hospitalization in the neonatal intensive care unit (NICU)
      2. Oxygen requirements in the nursery
      3. Respiratory conditions that required continuous positive airway pressure or endotracheal intubation
      4. Length of time on positive pressure ventilation

  5. Apnea
  6. Congenital heart defects that increase pulmonary blood flow
  7. When discharged after birth
 D. Review of Systems
  1. General: growth (poor weight gain may indicate cystic fibrosis)
  2. Respiratory: more than 6 to 10 upper respiratory infections per year, frequent lower respiratory tract infections, number of episodes of acute otitis media, sinusitis, asthma, bronchopulmonary dysplasia, viral croup, epiglottitis, pharyngitis, tonsillitis, peritonsillar abscess, retropharyngeal abscess, bacterial tracheitis, chronic cough, laryngomalacia, tracheomalacia, cystic fibrosis, pneumonia, bronchiolitis, tuberculosis, pertussis, pneumothorax
  3. Integumentary: atopic dermatitis
  4. Cardiovascular: congenital heart defects that increase pulmonary blood flow
  5. Immunity: allergic rhinitis, allergic angioedema
 E. Past Medical History
  1. Diagnosed respiratory conditions
  2. Growth failure
  3. Chronic cough
  4. Chest pain
  5. Cyanosis
 F. Immunization History
 G. Allergies
  1. Types
  2. Reactions
 H. Hospitalizations for Respiratory Conditions
  1. Date
  2. Diagnosis
  3. Length of stay
 I. Injuries
  1. Smoke inhalation
  2. Chemical inhalation
  3. Blunt chest trauma
 J. Current Medications
  1. Bronchodilators
  2. Corticosteroids
  3. Mast cell stabilizers
  4. Leukotriene receptor agonists
  5. Methylxanthines
  6. Expectorants
  7. Antihistamines
  8. Alternative/complimentary therapies
  9. Over-the-counter medications
  10. Include dose and frequency for each medication
 K. Family History
  1. Cystic fibrosis
  2. Atopy
  3. Asthma

    L. **Social History**
1. Exposure to second- or third-hand smoke
2. Exposure to allergens in home
3. Exposure to pollution
4. Does the child smoke?
5. Involvement in sports (include type of sport and frequency of participation)
6. Hobbies that involve respiratory exposure to chemical irritants
7. Recent immigration from country with high prevalence of tuberculosis
8. Homelessness

    M. **History of Present Illness**
1. Respiratory complaints
2. Fever
3. Cough
4. Sputum
5. Exercise intolerance
6. Chest pain
7. Growth failure
8. Ear pain
9. Headache, vomiting, abdominal pain

II. **Physical Examination**
    A. **Vital Signs**
    B. **Weight and Height; Plot on Growth Chart; Compare With Previous Measurements**
    C. **Inspection**
1. General appearance
2. Respiratory rate/effort/distress
3. Skin color
4. Apical impulse
5. Finger clubbing
6. Diaphoresis
7. Edema
8. Chest deformity

    D. **Auscultation**
1. Normal breath sounds
2. Adventitious breath sounds

    E. **Palpation**
1. Respiratory excursion
2. Fremitus
3. Regional lymph nodes

    F. **Percussion**
1. Indirect
2. Direct

RESPIRATORY SYSTEM: WRITE-UP

Use the space provided here to document all subjective and objective findings using the SOAP rubric.

Subjective—(historical information; chief complaint; history of present illness)

_____

_____

Objective—(vital signs, physical examination findings, results of laboratory and other diagnostic tests)

_____

_____

Assessment—(diagnosis [use ICD-10 codes]; other health issues that are identified)

_____

_____

Plan—(treatment, medications, therapies, teaching, referrals, follow-up care)

_____

_____

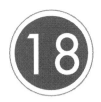

Assessment of the Cardiovascular System

CHAPTER OVERVIEW

The ability to obtain a thorough and complete cardiovascular history and physical assessment is a critical skill for the pediatric health care provider to possess. Knowledge of cardiac anatomy and physiology, normal vital signs for age, and the use of inspection, palpation, and auscultation techniques and maneuvers can help to formulate accurate differential diagnoses. Developmental approaches to the physical exam are important, especially for younger children.

Expected Learning Outcomes

After reading Chiocca, Advanced Pediatric Assessment, *Second Edition*, Chapter 18, the learner will be able to:

1. Demonstrate the ability to obtain an accurate and thorough cardiovascular health history for all pediatric age groups
2. Complete an accurate and thorough physical examination of the cardiovascular system for all pediatric age groups
3. Identify and differentiate normal and abnormal heart sounds in infants and children
4. Identify murmurs associated with pediatric cardiac defects
5. Demonstrate the ability to record all health assessment findings accurately and completely

Essential Terminology

Aortic valve—a cardiac valve that lies between the left ventricle and the aorta; has three leaflets; prevents blood from flowing from the aorta back into the left ventricle; one of the semilunar valves

Apex of the heart—the narrow, pointed, lowest portion of the heart; exact location in the chest depends on the child's age, size, or medical condition

Base of the heart—the broad upper portion of the heart

Bradycardia—abnormally slow heart rate; in children the normal heart rate is age dependent, thus definition of tachycardia will vary

Click—heart sound heard early in systole immediately following S_1(systolic ejection click); heard in children with lesions involving semilunar valves

Clubbing—a broad, convex appearance of the fingers and toes caused by chronic arterial desaturation

Congenital heart disease—one or more defects in the structure of the heart or great vessels that is present at birth

Critical congenital heart disease—a congenital cardiac defect that will require surgery or cardiac catheter-based treatment during the first year of life; includes seven specific congenital cardiac defects

Cyanosis—bluish color of the skin or mucous membranes caused by deoxygenated blood; can be central (visible on trunk, lips, tongue) or peripheral (seen on extremities, fingers, and toes)

Dextrocardia—a condition in which the heart is located in the middle or the right side of the chest; the heart may be rotated or a mirror image of a normally positioned heart

Diaphoresis—in children with cardiac disease, excessive sweating caused by a sympathetic nervous system response to increased cardiac demands and decreased cardiac output

Diastole—ventricular relaxation; causes the semilunar valves to close, preventing blood from flowing back into the ventricles

Diastolic murmur—a murmur that occurs between S_2 and S_1; best heard with the diaphragm of stethoscope at the left sternal border; always pathologic

Dyspnea—difficulty breathing

Edema—retention of interstitial fluid; etiology can be renal or cardiac; causes a swollen appearance first in dependent parts of body (e.g., lower extremities), then, as the problem progresses, over the entire body

Endocardium—the innermost layer that lines the four heart chambers and valves

Epicardium—the thin, outer muscular layer that covers the heart

Fetal circulation—the circulatory system of the fetus; which differs in several important ways from the postnatal circulation; in the fetus, the placenta is mainly responsible for oxygenating and filtering the blood, and there are four fetal shunts that permit blood to bypass the lungs

First heart sound (S_1)—the heart sound that marks the beginning of systole; it is generated by the closure of the atrioventricular valves; S_1 is synchronous with the apical pulse and is best heard at the apex or lower left sternal border

Fourth heart sound (S_4)—the heart sound heard immediately preceding the first heart sound (S_1); associated with atrial contraction and excessive flow across the atrioventricular valves; rare in children; always pathologic and suggests congestive heart failure

Gallop rhythm—tachycardia in combination with a normal S_1, S_2, and audible S_3 with or without an S_4; a pathologic finding due to overload such as congestive heart failure

Innocent murmur—a nonpathologic heart murmur

Intensity—the loudness of a turbulent blood flow through a heart valve or vessel (murmur); quantified in grades from I to VI

Location—auscultatory area where a heart sound is found

Mesocardia—a condition in which the heart is located in the midline of the chest

Midclavicular line (MCL)—an imaginary vertical line drawn on either side of the chest; begins at midclavicle and extends downward; used as a landmark to locate the apex of the heart and to assess liver size

Mitral valve—the cardiac valve that lies between the left atrium and left ventricle; the left atrioventricular valve

Myocardium—the thick, muscular, middle layer of the heart; responsible for contraction of the heart

Pallor—pale color of skin and mucous membranes

Palpitations—rapid, irregular heartbeat

Pericardial friction rub—a harsh, to-and-fro sound heard best at the lower left sternal border; caused by the heart rubbing against the pericardium; most common in the initial postoperative period after open heart surgery

Pericardium—the fibrous, double-walled sac that encases the heart and acts as a protective cover

Point of maximal impulse (PMI)—farthest point from the sternum where the cardiac impulse can be palpated; the location varies according to the child's age

Precordium—the area of the anterior chest that covers the heart and great vessels

Pulmonary artery—the artery that carries venous blood from the right ventricle to the lungs

Pulmonic valve—a cardiac valve that lies between the right ventricle and the pulmonary artery; has three leaflets; prevents blood from flowing from the pulmonary artery back into the right ventricle; one of the semilunar valves

Quality—a term used in describing cardiac murmur; for example, "blowing" quality

Rate—the number of heart beats per minute; heart sounds are also auscultated apically and compared to the rate of the radial pulse to assess for synchronicity

Rhythm—the regularity of the heart beat

Second heart sound (S_2)—the heart sound that marks the beginning of diastole; it is generated by the closure of the semilunar valves; best heard at the upper left sternal border with the diaphragm of the stethoscope

Semilunar valves—the collective name for two heart valves, the aortic and pulmonic valves; each has three leaflets that act to prevent blood from flowing back into the ventricles

Syncope—transient loss of consciousness and muscle tone; has various etiologies

Systole—ventricular contraction; opens the semilunar valves to allow blood into the great arteries

Systolic murmur—a murmur that occurs between S_1 and S_2; the most common type of murmur heard in children

Tachycardia—abnormally rapid heart rate; in children the normal heart rate is age dependent, thus definition of tachycardia will vary

Third heart sound (S_3)—a heart sound caused by ventricular dilation or decreased ventricular compliance; sounds like "Kentucky" on auscultation; often an early sign of heart failure

Thrill—a visible or palpable vibratory sensation on the chest caused by turbulent blood flow

Timing—an technique used to assess cardiac murmurs that involves describing when in the S_1–S_2 cycle a murmur is heard; helps to define the etiology of a murmur

Transmission—the movement of heart sounds to another anatomic location; for example, a systolic murmur auscultated in the neck region

Tricuspid valve—the cardiac valve that lies between the right atrium and right ventricle; the right atrioventricular valve

CRITICAL THINKING EXERCISES

Short-Answer Critical Thinking Exercises

1. Discuss fetal circulation in detail. Trace the flow of blood beginning at the placenta. What role do in utero fetal shunts play in understanding the pathophysiology and presenting time frame of cyanotic and acyanotic congenital heart defects?
2. Discuss the transition from fetal circulation that occurs when the umbilical cord is clamped and the infant takes the first breath of life.
3. Describe normal anatomy of the heart and outline blood circulation through the heart and lungs.
4. What are some risk factors for congenital heart defects?
5. Discuss the neonatal screening recommendations for critical congenital heart disease using pulse oximetry.
6. When obtaining the cardiac health history in a child, what are some important questions to ask?
7. Describe a complete pediatric heart assessment. Discuss the systematic approach that should be routinely followed so that no cardiovascular assessments are missed.
8. When conducting the pediatric physical examination, what extracardiac physical findings can yield information about a child's cardiovascular status?
9. Compare and contrast innocent and pathologic murmurs. What are the specific characteristics of pathologic murmurs?
10. What is the difference between a systolic and diastolic murmur?

Critical Thinking Case Study Exercises

Exercise 1

Sarah is an 8-month-old infant brought to the clinic by her parents, who say they are concerned because Sarah does not seem to be "growing normally."

Sarah's mother states that Sarah's first cousin, born 1 week after her, weighs 3 pounds more than she does. Upon further questioning by the health care provider, Sarah's parents report that she usually falls asleep approximately halfway through her bottle feedings and appears "tired and sweaty" when this happens.

1. What other historical data should the provider obtain?
2. What should be included in Sarah's cardiovascular exam? What is the systematic approach that should be taken to ensure a complete assessment?
3. Sarah has a grade III/VI regurgitant murmur on auscultation, but no palpable thrill. What is her likely diagnosis? Is this an innocent or pathologic murmur?
4. How does Sarah's history relate to the history that her mother reports?
5. Does Sarah require a referral?

Exercise 2

Lucia is a 15-month-old girl who presents to the clinic in October for a regular health maintenance examination. Lucia was diagnosed with total anomalous pulmonary venous return (TAPVR) without obstruction at age 2 months and underwent surgical repair a month later. Her past medical history is otherwise unremarkable, and she is not on any medications. Lucia was last seen by the pediatric cardiologist at age 12 months. Currently, her weight and height are in the 50th percentile, and her developmental assessment is within normal limits. Her physical examination reveals a well-nourished, active toddler.

1. What should Lucia's review of systems include?
2. Discuss examples of cardiac, pulmonary, gastrointestinal, and neurologic physical assessment findings that would be of concern if observed while examining Lucia.
3. Should Lucia receive the recommended immunizations for her age group? Why or why not?
4. Given the time of year, what should be recommended for Lucia, given her age and cardiac history?

Exercise 3

Juan is a 6-year-old boy who presents to the clinic accompanied by his mother. Juan's family has recently emigrated from Mexico. His mother states that Juan had only episodic health care while in Mexico, and she is unsure of his immunization status. Juan's mother states that he has never been as active as other children, and now that he is in school in the United States, she received a note from the gym teacher stating that Juan cannot complete what the other children are doing without frequent rest periods.

1. What should Juan's review of systems include?
2. What historical questions should the provider ask that are specific to his presenting complaint?
3. Is Juan's immunization history relevant to his potential diagnosis?
4. What objective data are essential to obtain?
5. What objective findings would be indicative of cardiac disease in Juan?

Exercise 4

Paul is a 12-year-old boy whose parents bring him to the emergency room with complaints of chest pain. Paul's father states that the chest pain has occurred on and off since Paul started playing baseball. His mother is clearly frightened and states she is concerned that Paul is having a heart attack, as her father died 20 years ago of a myocardial infarction at age 65 years. The family history is otherwise unremarkable for cardiovascular conditions. Paul is not exposed to secondhand smoke. Currently, Paul's color is pink and he is in no apparent distress. His vital signs are: temperature 97.6°F (36.4°C); heart rate 84 bpm and regular; respirations 20; blood pressure 106/62. Paul's weight and height are in the 50th percentile.

1. What other historical data are important to gather for this child?
2. What specific questions should be asked to differentiate between a pathologic and nonpathologic cause of Paul's chest pain?
3. Are most episodes of chest pain in children cardiac in nature?
4. What should Paul's physical examination include?

Refer to Figure 18.1 in the textbook and label the cardiac anatomy in the illustration that follows.

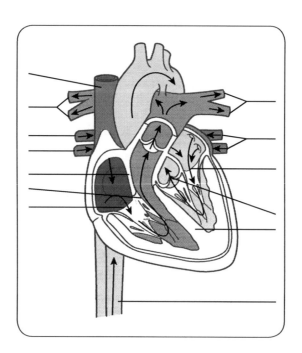

Refer to Figure 18.2 in the textbook and label fetal cardiac anatomy and circulatory blood flow in the illustration that follows.

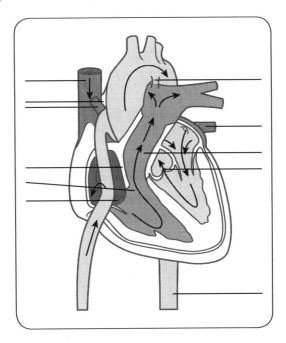

Refer to Figures 18.3 and 18.9 in the textbook and label the point of maximum impulse and anatomic locations where systolic murmurs are best heard.

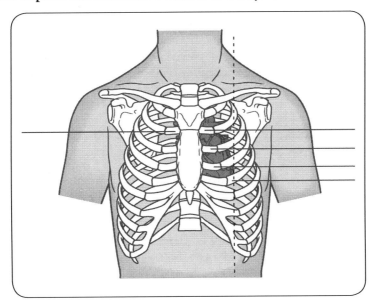

REVIEW QUESTIONS

1. Which of the following maternal conditions is associated with congenital heart disease?

   a. Maternal rubella
   b. Type 1 diabetes

    c. Syncope

    d. Gonorrhea

2. The congenital heart defect depicted in this image is:

    a. Patent ductus arteriosus

    b. Coarctation of the aorta

    c. Ventricular septal defect

    d. Atrial septal defect

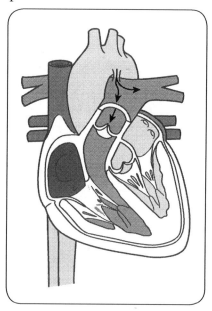

3. Which of the following correctly describes the steps in the systematic approach to cardiac auscultation in infants and children?

    a. Identify S_1, S_2, then the splitting of S_2, then S_3 and S_4

    b. Identify S_1, S_2, then auscultate for any murmurs, then listen for S_3 and S_4

    c. Identify S_1, S_2, then the splitting of S_2, then auscultate for any murmurs

    d. Identify all heart sounds at once

4. The optimal location for auscultation of the murmur associated with an atrial septal defect is:

    a. The upper left sternal border

    b. The lower left sternal border

    c. The upper right sternal border

    d. The lower right sternal border

5. When conducting a physical examination on a 5-day-old neonate, which of the following findings suggests coarctation of the aorta?

    a. Bounding pulses in all four extremities

    b. Gallop rhythm

    c. Higher blood pressure in the right arm than in the right leg

    d. Diastolic rumble

6. During the physical examination of a 1-year-old child, the examiner notes a thrill in the left lower sternal border. The most likely etiology of this finding is:

    a. Ventricular septal defect
    b. Aortic stenosis
    c. Arterial stenosis
    d. Pulmonary stenosis

7. A cardiac murmur that is moderately loud with no palpable thrill is classified as:

    a. Grade II
    b. Grade III
    c. Grade V
    d. Grade VI

8. Which of the following findings seen in adults with congestive heart failure is rarely seen in children with this diagnosis?

    a. Eyelid edema
    b. Facial edema
    c. Abdominal ascites
    d. Pitting edema

9. The PMI in children is located:

    a. At the intersection of the fifth intercostal space and the left MCL
    b. At the intersection of the fourth intercostal space and the left MCL
    c. At the fifth intercostal space just lateral to the left nipple
    d. At the fourth intercostal space just medial to the left nipple

10. Which of the following assessment maneuvers can be helpful in differentiating between a pathologic and an innocent murmur in a child?

    a. Encouraging inspiration to clarify the right-sided lesions, such as pulmonary stenosis or tricuspid regurgitation
    b. Encouraging inspiration to decrease venous return to make the ejection click of pulmonary stenosis louder
    c. Asking the child or teen to lie prone for 30 seconds to assess intensity of innocent murmurs
    d. Asking the child or teen to exhale quickly to evaluate whether the murmur increases or decreases in intensity

11. A nonsedentary adolescent with a body mass index within normal limits complains of exercise intolerance during gym class. The health care provider should conduct a cardiovascular examination with which of the following differential diagnoses in mind?

    a. Heart failure
    b. Stroke
    c. Mitral valve prolapse
    d. Still's murmur

12. Which of the following correctly describes the quality of the murmur heard with a mitral valve prolapse?

   a. Gallop rhythm
   b. Midsystolic click
   c. Loud in midprecordium
   d. Ejection click

13. Which of the following parts of a child's perinatal history are red flags for congenital heart disease?

   a. Large for gestational age
   b. Cyanosis at birth
   c. Formula intolerance
   d. Meconium-stained amniotic fluid

14. In children, the second heart sound (S_2) is best heard:

   a. At the upper left sternal border with the diaphragm of the stethoscope
   b. At the lower left sternal border with the diaphragm of the stethoscope
   c. At the upper left sternal border with the bell of the stethoscope
   d. At the lower left sternal border with the bell of the stethoscope

15. Physiologic splitting of the second heart sound (S_2):

   a. Can occur with respiration and is normal
   b. Occurs with ventricular systole and is generated by the closure of the arterioventricular valves
   c. Is abnormal and is associated with pathologic conditions that cause ventricular dilation
   d. Is rare in children, always pathologic and suggests congestive heart failure

16. When assessing the pulse rate in children, it should be counted for:

   a. 15 seconds
   b. 30 seconds
   c. 45 seconds
   d. 60 seconds

17. It is important to auscultate lung sounds as part of the cardiac assessment in children in order to assess for the presence of:

   a. Pulmonary flow murmurs
   b. Rales or wheezes, which may indicate pulmonary congestion due to heart failure
   c. Systemic hypertension caused by coarctation of the aorta
   d. Pulmonary ejection murmurs

18. A gallop rhythm is caused by:

   a. Fever
   b. Fear

c. Normal variant

d. Volume overload

19. In a child with congenital heart disease, tachypnea accompanied by tachycardia may be a sign of:

    a. Left-sided heart failure

    b. Right-sided heart failure

    c. Acute rheumatic fever

    d. Polycythemia

20. A 5-year-old child with congenital heart disease has a palpable spleen. This is most likely due to:

    a. Congestive heart failure

    b. Bacterial endocarditis

    c. Splenic sequestration crisis

    d. This is a normal finding

SAMPLE DOCUMENTATION: ASSESSMENT OF THE CARDIOVASCULAR SYSTEM

Patient Name _____ Date of Birth_____ Date_____
Gender_____

I. **Health History**
   A. **Prenatal History**
      1. Maternal health history
         a. Maternal diabetes, systemic lupus erythematosus
         b. Infections (e.g., rubella, cytomegalovirus, herpes, coxsackievirus B)
         c. Medications (e.g., warfarin, lithium, phenytoin, nonsteroidal anti-inflammatory drugs [NSAIDs], amphetamines)
         d. Alcohol and recreational drug use
      2. Diagnosis of congenital heart defects in utero
   B. **Perinatal History**
      1. Fetal distress
      2. Hypoxia
      3. Cyanosis at birth requiring oxygen
      4. Prematurity
      5. Apgar scores
   C. **Postnatal History**
      1. Oxygen requirements in the nursery
      2. Respiratory or cardiac distress that required endotracheal intubation?
      3. Congenital heart disease diagnosed at birth (type)
      4. Neonatal course (e.g., cardiac catheterization, surgery; hospitalization in NICU or surgical heart unit; when discharged after birth)
   D. **Review of Systems**
      1. General
      2. Growth
      3. Integumentary
      4. Cardiovascular

    5. Respiratory

    6. Neurologic

    7. Hematologic

    8. Endocrine

    9. Infectious diseases

    10. Immunologic

    11. Rheumatologic

    12. Gastrointestinal

    13. Genitourinary

E. **Past Medical History**

    1. Diagnosed congenital heart lesion

    2. Growth failure

    3. Exercise intolerance

    4. Respiratory complaints

    5. Poor feeding in infancy

    6. Chest pain

    7. Syncope

    8. Joint symptoms

    9. Neurologic symptoms

    10. Cyanosis

    11. Hypertension

    12. Hyperlipidemia

    13. Congestive heart failure

    14. Cardiomyopathy

F. **Immunization History**

G. **Past Surgical History**

    1. Cardiac surgery (type, dates, cardiac lesion, child's postoperative course)

H. **Family History**

    1. Congenital heart disease

    2. Sudden, unexplained death of first-degree relative

    3. Arrhythmias

    4. Early myocardial infarction (before age 50)

    5. Hyperlipidemia

    6. Hypertension

    7. Obesity

    8. Genetic syndromes

    9. Parental consanguinity

I. **Social History**

    1. Involvement in sports (type of sport and frequency of participation)

    2. Use of recreational drugs

    3. Consumption of caffeinated drinks

J. **Medications**

    1. Name of drug, dose, and frequency

    2. Medications taken for cardiovascular conditions or that may have cardiac side effects (e.g., digoxin, diuretics, angiotensin-converting enzyme inhibitors, beta blockers, antihypertensives, antibiotics [rheumatic heart disease]).

K. History of Present Illness
1. Respiratory complaints
2. Exercise intolerance
3. Cyanosis
4. Syncope
5. Palpitations
6. Chest pain
7. Edema
8. Growth failure
9. Joint symptoms
10. Neurologic symptoms

II. Physical Examination
A. Vital Signs
B. Weight and Height; Plot on Growth Chart; Compare With Previous Measurements
C. Inspection
1. General appearance
2. Respiratory effort
3. Skin color
4. Apical impulse
5. Clubbing
6. Diaphoresis
7. Edema
8. Jugular venous distention
9. Diaphoresis
10. Chest deformity
11. Extracardiac anomalies
D. Palpation
1. Precordial activity
2. Apical impulse
3. PMI
4. Thrills
5. Peripheral pulses
6. Liver
7. Spleen
E. Auscultation
1. Heart sounds
   a. Heart rate and rhythm
   b. Systole and diastole
   c. S_1 and S_2
   d. Extra heart sounds
      i. Clicks
      ii. Murmurs
2. Friction rub
3. Lungs

CARDIOVASCULAR SYSTEM: WRITE-UP

Use the space provided here to document all subjective and objective findings using the SOAP rubric.

Subjective—(historical information; chief complaint; history of present illness)

_____

_____

Objective—(vital signs, physical examination findings, results of laboratory and other diagnostic tests)

_____

_____

Assessment—(diagnosis [use ICD-10 codes]; other health issues that are identified)

_____

_____

Plan—(treatment, medications, therapies, teaching, referrals, follow-up care)

_____

_____

Assessment of the Abdomen and Regional Lymphatics

CHAPTER OVERVIEW

This chapter helps to solidify the skills needed to perform an accurate age- and developmentally appropriate examination of the abdomen, to recognize deviations from normal, and to accurately record assessment findings.

Expected Learning Outcomes

After reading Chiocca, *Advanced Pediatric Assessment, Second Edition*, Chapter 19, the learner will be able to:

1. Obtain a thorough and accurate pediatric abdominal history
2. Examine the abdomen using inspection, auscultation, percussion, and palpation, and distinguish normal and abnormal findings
3. Analyze historical and physical assessment findings related to the abdomen and use these data to make accurate assessments and diagnoses
4. Accurately record history and physical assessment findings related to assessment of the abdomen

Essential Terminology

Costovertebral angle—the area below the angle that is formed by the 12th rib and the vertebral column; the kidneys lie directly below this area

Diastasis recti—a midline bulge between separated rectus muscles

Hepatomegaly—enlarged liver

Scaphoid—sunken abdominal wall; occurs with severe malnutrition or in neonates with congenital defects that involve the abdominal contents

Splenomegaly—enlarged spleen

Tympany—the most common percussion note throughout the abdomen in children; caused by gas in the stomach, small bowel, and colon; the sound is high-pitched, musical, and drum-like

Label the anatomic structures indicated on these illustrations.

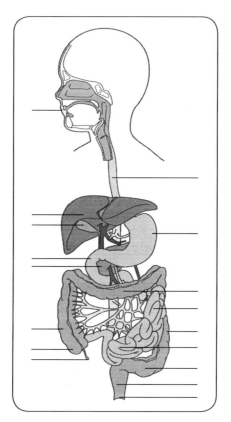

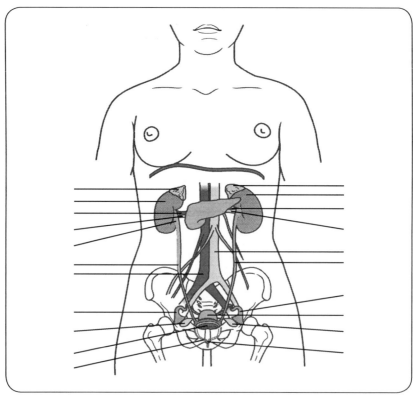

CRITICAL THINKING EXERCISES

Short-Answer Critical Thinking Exercises

1. Describe the procedure for examining the abdomen in infants, children, and adolescents. How is modesty maintained?
2. State the sequence of assessment techniques when examining the abdomen in children and why it differs from other body systems.
3. Discuss some techniques that can facilitate examination of the abdomen in young children.
4. Name the contents of each quadrant of the abdomen.

   a. Right upper quadrant (RUQ) _____
   b. Right lower quadrant (RLQ) _____
   c. Left lower quadrant (LLQ) _____
   d. Left upper quadrant (LUQ) _____

5. Which organs can be easily palpated in a child's abdomen? Which cannot be easily palpated?
6. Discuss the differential diagnoses of abdominal pain based on abdominal location.
7. Discuss the difference between light and deep palpation and the indications for each.
8. List and describe the normal percussion notes when assessing the abdomen. Do they differ according to age? How?

Critical Thinking Case Study Exercises

Exercise 1

Mavis is an uncooperative, obese toddler who is kicking and crying during her well-child exam. Her mother is asking that you defer the examination of her abdomen, but the history reveals that Mavis moves her bowels only one to two times per week, and had a red, itchy area in the suprapubic region.

1. What other parts of Mavis's history would you like to know?
2. What are some techniques you can use to get Mavis to cooperate with the exam?
3. What are you looking for in your exam of Mavis?

Exercise 2

Mason is an 18-month-old toddler, brought to the clinic by his mother. Mason's mother states that he appears to have frequent stomach aches and he strains and cries when trying to move his bowels. Upon auscultation of his abdomen, you note that he has normal bowel sounds, and palpation of his abdomen reveals a firm sausage-like mass, palpable in the LLQ.

1. What questions regarding Mason's past medical history would you like to know?
2. What other questions would you ask Mason's mother to regarding the reason for seeking health care?

3. Are there any other physical assessments that should be done?
4. What are your differential diagnoses for Mason?

Exercise 3

The parents of a 3-week-old male infant, Gio, bring him to the clinic stating that he has been crying inconsolably, appears famished, but when he breast-feeds, he vomits all that he consumed shortly after nursing. His parents say that now, the vomit "shoots out." Upon physical examination, one finding is a palpable, olive-shaped mass in Gio's RUQ.

1. What other historical data need to be obtained? Include past and current histories.
2. What other physical assessments should be done? Be specific, and consider Gio's age.
3. What are your differential diagnoses for Gio?

Exercise 4

John is a 15-year-old boy whose parents bring him to the clinic with complaints of vomiting and generalized abdominal pain for the past 48 hours. Now the abdominal pain is localized to the RLQ, and John is guarding his abdomen.

1. What other parts of John's history would you like to know?
2. What additional physical examination would you do?
3. What condition do you suspect?

REVIEW QUESTIONS

1. Select the correct sequence of techniques used during an examination of a child's abdomen.

   a. Percussion, inspection, palpation, auscultation
   b. Inspection, palpation, percussion, auscultation
   c. Inspection, auscultation, percussion, palpation
   d. Auscultation, inspection, palpation, percussion

2. When percussing a child's abdomen, you note tympany. This is indicative of the presence of:

   a. Fluid
   b. Air
   c. Feces
   d. Hepatomegaly

3. When inspecting the child's abdomen, the examiner notes a midline muscular separation with bulging as the child cries. This finding is a(n):

   a. Umbilical hernia
   b. Inguinal hernia

   c. Omphalocele

   d. Diastasis recti

4. A 10-month-old infant is brought to the clinic with complaints of cough and rhinorrhea. When auscultating the child's lungs, you note a large, bulging umbilical mass. The mass is easily reducible but increases when the child cries. This assessment finding is a(n):

   a. Inguinal hernia

   b. Umbilical hernia

   c. Gastroschisis

   d. Omphalocele

5. The iliopsoas test is used to identify:

   a. Splenic enlargement

   b. Costovertebral tenderness

   c. Intra-abdominal inflammation

   d. Decreased peristalsis or intestinal activity

6. When auscultating bowel sounds in an infant or a young child, it is essential to use a pediatric stethoscope because:

   a. A stethoscope diaphragm that is too large may also encompass lung sounds, confusing the clinical picture

   b. A stethoscope diaphragm that is too large may also encompass vascular sounds, confusing the clinical picture

   c. A stethoscope diaphragm that is too large may cause pain in a small infant if pressure is applied during auscultation

   d. A stethoscope diaphragm that is too large may decrease the child's cooperation

7. Decreased hepatic enzyme function in children from birth until age 3 to 4 years causes:

   a. Short drug half-lives

   b. Long drug half-lives

   c. Physiologic jaundice

   d. Hypoglycemia

8. The stomach capacity in a neonate is approximately:

   a. 30 mL

   b. 60 mL

   c. 90 mL

   d. 120 mL

9. A dull percussion note at or beyond the anterior axillary line on the left indicates:

   a. Hepatomegaly

   b. Splenomegaly

    c. A normal finding
    d. A fibrotic spleen

10. Assessment for renal tenderness should be performed with the child:

    a. Lying supine
    b. Lying prone
    c. In a side-lying position
    d. Sitting upright

11. Indirect percussion can be used to detect:

    a. Costovertebral tenderness
    b. Abdominal masses
    c. Rebound tenderness
    d. Hepatomegaly

12. The LLQ contains the:

    a. Left ureter
    b. Pancreas (body)
    c. Stomach
    d. Liver (left lobe)

13. The percussion note that is normally heard over a child's stomach is:

    a. Dull
    b. Tympany
    c. Resonance
    d. Hyperactive

14. A firm, olive-like mass palpable in the RUQ of a 3-week-old infant is likely a(n):

    a. Fecal mass
    b. Pyloric stenosis
    c. Umbilical hernia
    d. Inguinal hernia

15. Infants and toddlers have a protuberant abdomen due to:

    a. Increased pancreatic enzyme activity
    b. Weak abdominal musculature
    c. More abdominal subcutaneous tissue
    d. Decreased hepatic enzyme function

16. A young child's kidney is more susceptible to trauma because:

    a. Until age 5 years, kidneys rupture more easily
    b. More of the kidney is exposed because of the thin abdominal wall
    c. A proportionately larger abdomen in young children
    d. The urinary bladder capacity varies

17. Which of the following is an appropriate response by the provider to a 30-month-old child who is resistant to the abdominal exam?

    a. Inspect only; auscultate and palpate only if necessary
    b. Ask the child to describe the symptoms in more detail
    c. Ask the child if he or she would like to listen to the stomach through the stethoscope and press on the stomach with his or her own hands
    d. Defer the exam

18. Which of the following findings in the child's prenatal history is relevant when conducting the abdominal assessment?

    a. Maternal oligohydramnios
    b. Amount of maternal weight gain
    c. Perinatal asphyxia
    d. Timing of the first meconium stool

19. The RLQ contains the:

    a. Liver (right lobe)
    b. Pancreas
    c. Ascending colon
    d. Cecum

20. The provider palpates the child's abdomen slowly and deeply away from an area of tenderness, then quickly removes the palpating hand. The child experiences pain when the palpating hand is removed quickly. This describes:

    a. Light palpation
    b. Rebound tenderness
    c. Deep palpation
    d. Costovertebral tenderness

SAMPLE DOCUMENTATION: ASSESSMENT OF THE ABDOMEN AND REGIONAL LYMPHATICS

Patient Name _____ Date of Birth_____ Date_____
Gender_____

  I. **Health History**
    A. **Reason for Seeking Health care** (e.g. routine well-child examination; abdominal complaint)
      1. Past medical history
        a. Prenatal, birth, neonatal histories
        b. Chronic health conditions related to the abdomen
        c. Obesity
        d. Past hospitalizations (e.g., abdominal injuries or infections)
        e. Surgical history
        f. Family medical history (e.g., irritable bowel disease, Crohn's disease, lactose intolerance, or sickle cell disease)

      g. Current medications
      h. Immunization history
      i. Review of systems
   2. Nutritional history
   3. Elimination patterns
   4. Social history (e.g., recurrent abdominal pain)

II. Physical Examination
   A. Inspection of the Abdomen
   B. Auscultation of the Abdomen
   C. Percussion of the Abdomen
   D. Palpation of the Abdomen
      1. Light palpation
      2. Deep palpation

ASSESSMENT OF THE ABDOMEN AND REGIONAL LYMPHATICS: WRITE-UP

Use the space provided here to document all subjective and objective findings using the SOAP rubric.

Subjective—(historical information; chief complaint; history of present illness)

_____

_____

Objective—(vital signs, physical examination findings, results of laboratory and other diagnostic tests)

_____

_____

Assessment—(diagnosis [use ICD-10 codes]; other health issues that are identified)

_____

_____

Plan—(treatment, medications, therapies, teaching, referrals, follow-up care)

_____

_____

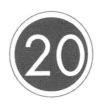

Assessment of the Reproductive and Genitourinary Systems

CHAPTER OVERVIEW

Assessment of the reproductive system can provoke a great deal of anxiety for the child or adolescent, the parent, and the provider. This chapter assists in gaining the skills to facilitate obtaining an accurate and complete pediatric genitourinary assessment in children of all ages.

Expected Learning Outcomes

After reading Chiocca, *Advanced Pediatric Assessment, Second Edition*, Chapter 20, the learner will be able to:

1. Obtain a thorough and accurate pediatric genitourinary history
2. Demonstrate sensitivity and maintain privacy when conducting the pediatric genitourinary history and physical examination
3. Examine the male genitalia and abdomen using inspection and palpation, and distinguish normal and abnormal findings
4. Examine the female genitalia and abdomen using inspection and palpation, and distinguish normal and abnormal findings
5. Perform an accurate pelvic and bimanual examination on an adolescent female
6. Analyze historical and physical assessment findings related to the genitourinary tract and use these data to make accurate assessments and diagnoses
7. Accurately record history and physical assessment findings related to assessment of the genitourinary tract

Essential Terminology

Cervix—the entry to the uterus; allows menstrual blood and fetus to pass from the uterus into the vagina

Clitoris—a small structure composed of erectile tissue, located just below the mons pubis in females

Fallopian tubes—two long, muscular tubes having a funnel-shaped opening at one end that extends close to or over the ovaries; projections at the fimbriated end pull the ovum into the fallopian tube after it is released from the ovary

Hymen—a fold of mucous membrane that partially covers the vaginal orifice

Menarche—the onset of menstruation

Mons pubis—the most visible part of the female external genitalia; an area of adipose tissue covered with skin; after a girl reaches puberty, the mons pubis is covered with coarse, curly pubic hair

Labia majora—prominent, longitudinal skin folds situated in the perineum

Labia minora—two hairless folds of tissue that lie between the labia majora and the urethral *and* vaginal orifices

Ovaries—two almond-shaped organs that produce the female hormones and normally release one mature ovum a month

Uterus—a muscular organ in the female reproductive tract that houses the fertilized ovum, which becomes the embryo and then the fetus

Vagina—a tubular, muscular structure in females that acts as a passageway for menstrual blood, facilitates sexual intercourse, and serves as the passageway for the infant during childbirth

Vaginitis—inflammation of the vagina

Vestibule—the area covered by the labia minora

Vulva—the collective term for the female external genitalia

Label the anatomic structures indicated on these illustrations.

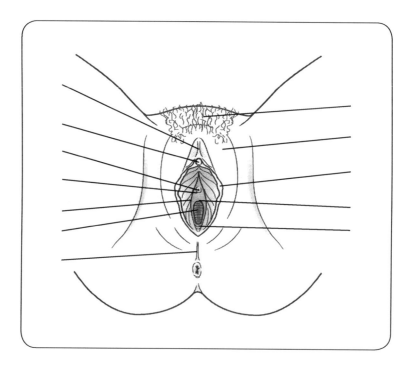

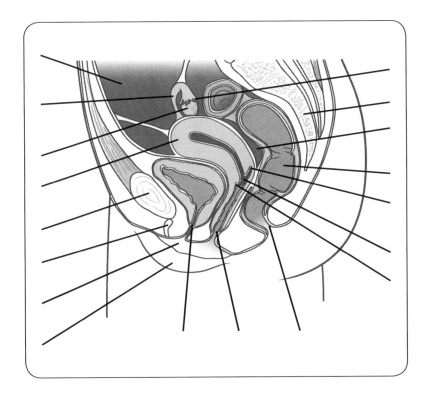

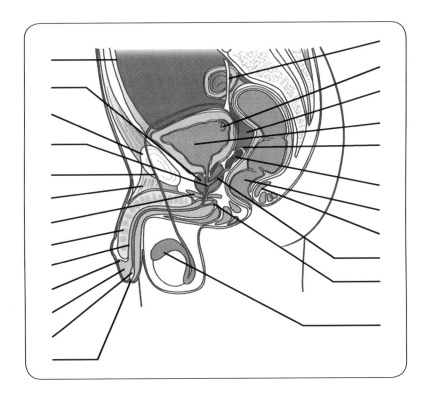

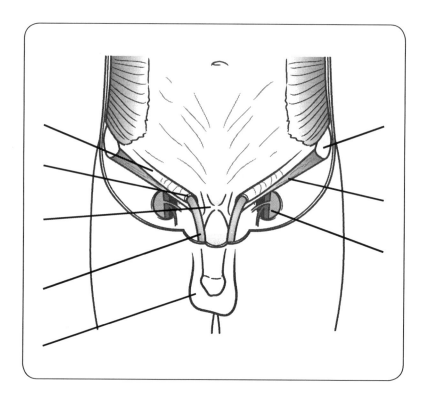

CRITICAL THINKING EXERCISES

Short-Answer Critical Thinking Exercises

1. Explain the stages of sexual maturation for both females and males.
2. What factors could affect the onset of puberty in a child? Discuss both delayed and early-onset puberty.
3. Discuss some communication strategies that are necessary when examining the genitourinary area in a child or adolescent. Be specific for each age and developmental stage.
4. What are the indications for a pelvic examination in an adolescent girl?
5. Describe the steps involved in conducting a pelvic exam on an adolescent girl.
6. At what age should an adolescent female begin breast self-exams?
7. At what age should an adolescent male begin testicular self-exams?
8. Discuss the difference between retractile testes and cryptorchidism. How are they distinguished? At what point would the child require a referral?

Critical Thinking Case Study Exercises

Exercise 1

Describe the components of the well-child genitourinary exam for each age group and gender that appears in the following table.

AGE GROUP	FEMALE	MALE
Infant		
Toddler		
Preschool child		
School-aged child		
Prepubescent adolescent		
Postpubescent adolescent		

Exercise 2

A 5-month-old boy, Zach, is brought to the emergency room by his parents. They say that he has frequent diaper rashes and they think that Zach's nanny does not change his diaper frequently enough. Over the past 2 days, they have noticed that the tip of Zach's penis is erythematous and edematous, and they are worried that it will affect Zach's ability to urinate.

1. What other historical data should you obtain?
2. What should the physical examination entail?
3. What is your differential diagnosis?

Exercise 3

A 15–year-old girl is at the clinic for her annual health screening visit. She has no significant past medical history. You have asked the mother to step out while you collect historical data that may be sensitive. Use the space that follows to list the questions you would ask, and information you would gather from the chart and American Academy of Pediatrics (AAP) periodicity table (see Chapter 6, *Advanced Pediatric Assessment, Second Edition*) to determine whether this adolescent girl needs a pelvic exam or Pap smear, or both.

Exercise 4

Tim is a 17-year-old boy with no significant past medical history, who is at the clinic for both a school and a sports physical. He has not had a "checkup" since he entered high school. Use the space that follows to list the historical questions you would ask that focus on the genitourinary system, and information you would gather from the chart and AAP periodicity table (see Chapter 6, *Advanced Pediatric Assessment, Second Edition*) to determine what type of physical examination you need to do.

REVIEW QUESTIONS

1. A child with sparse, pigmented, long, straight pubic hair, mainly along the labia or base of the penis would be considered to be in Tanner stage:

   a. I
   b. II
   c. III
   d. IV

2. While examining a 3-year-old child for a well-child visit, labial adhesions are noted. This finding is the result of:

   a. The labia minora being fused as a result of being in a hypoestrogenized state
   b. The labia minora being fused as a result of repeated vulvovaginitis
   c. The labia minora being fused as a result of a congenital defect
   d. The labia minora being fused as a result of sexual abuse

3. The first signs of puberty in girls are:

   a. Menarche and pubarche
   b. Breast development and the growth of pubic hair
   c. Growth spurt and menarche
   d. Breast development and menarche

4. Which of the following may enhance the cooperation and alleviate anxiety of a young child during a genitourinary exam?

   a. Ask the parent to step out of the room
   b. Conduct the exam first so the child does not have to anticipate it during the entire visit
   c. Examine the child while he or she is lying supine on the parent's lap
   d. Examine the child while he or she is restrained by a medical assistant

5. A pelvic examination is indicated for which one of the following adolescent girls?

   a. A 16-year-old girl who is sexually active
   b. A 17 year-old girl with amenorrhea
   c. A healthy 18-year-old who is not sexually active
   d. A 16-year-old girl with a vaginal yeast infection

6. Which of the following is **not** an indication for a pelvic examination in an adolescent female?

   a. Persistent vaginal discharge
   b. Abnormal vaginal bleeding
   c. Amenorrhea
   d. Polyuria

7. The clinical finding that is most indicative of testicular torsion is:

   a. Absence of the cremasteric reflex
   b. Positive transillumination of the scrotum
   c. Acute onset of excruciating testicular pain
   d. Dysuria

8. Mike is an infant in the clinic for his 6-month health maintenance visit. The examiner cannot palpate the right testicle. What should be the *next* step?

   a. Try to search for the testicle along the inguinal canal and try to milk it down into the scrotum
   b. Examine the medical record to see if any other examiner has been able to palpate Mike's right testicle
   c. Elicit the cremasteric reflex
   d. Place an order for an ultrasound of the scrotum

9. The condition in which the urethral meatus is located on the dorsal surface of the penis is:

   a. Hypospadias
   b. Epispadias
   c. Balanitis
   d. Chordee

10. Upon physical examination of a 2-year-old, uncircumcised male, you observe that the foreskin is retracted and slightly erythematous. The glans is swollen. Because of the swelling, you are unable to return the foreskin to its original position. This describes:

    a. Phimosis
    b. Paraphimosis
    c. Balanitis
    d. Urethritis

11. A 2-month-old baby boy presents with erythema and edema of the glans. Your differential diagnosis includes:

    a. Priapism
    b. Balanitis
    c. Chordee
    d. Epididymitis

12. The tissue between the labia minora may be fused as a result of being in a hypoestrogenized state, a condition known as:

    a. Labial adhesions
    b. Vulvovaginitis
    c. Chemical urethritis
    d. Lichen sclerosis

13. Pubic hair that appears as an inverted triangle, extending along the labia majora, and onto the medial surface of the thighs is Tanner stage:

   a. II
   b. III
   c. IV
   d. V

14. According to the American Academy of Pediatrics, at what age should an adolescent girl be screened for cervical cancer?

   a. 16 years
   b. 18 years
   c. 20 years
   d. 21 years

15. Which of the following statements is correct regarding the timing of menarche?

   a. It occurs approximately 2 years after the appearance of breast buds
   b. It occurs approximately 2 years after the appearance of pubic hair
   c. It occurs approximately 1 year after the appearance of pubic hair
   d. It occurs approximately 1 year before the appearance of axillary hair

16. Retractile testes are within normal limits until age:

   a. 6 months
   b. 1 year
   c. 3 years
   d. Puberty

17. In a male with an enlarged scrotum, which of the following assessment techniques can be helpful in differentiating inguinal hernia from hydrocele?

   a. Palpating the scrotal contents
   b. Transillumination of the scrotum
   c. Asking the boy to squat, then inspecting the scrotum
   d. Inspecting the scrotum for rugae

18. A small amount of whitish, odorless, mucoid discharge in the prepubertal girl is likely:

   a. Physiologic leukorrhea
   b. Vaginal candidiasis
   c. Foreign body in the vagina
   d. *Chlamydia trachomatis*

19. Cryptorchidism is more common in:

   a. Infants with hypospadias
   b. Infants with vesicoureteral reflux
   c. Preterm infants
   d. Ambulatory infants

20. The breast bud stage in which the breast and nipple elevate as a small mound, and the areola widens describes Tanner stage:

    a. I
    b. II
    c. III
    d. IV

SAMPLE DOCUMENTATION: FEMALE GENITOURINARY ASSESSMENT

Patient Name _____ Date of Birth_____ Date _____
Gender_____

I. Health History
   A. **Reason for Seeking Health Care** (e.g., routine well-child examination; genitourinary complaint)
      1. Past medical history
         a. Prenatal, birth, neonatal histories
         b. Congenital anomalies affecting the genitourinary tract (see Box 20.1, *Advanced Pediatric Assessment, Second Edition*)
         c. Past hospitalizations (e.g., genitourinary injuries or infections)
         d. Surgical history
         e. Family medical history (see Box 20.2, *Advanced Pediatric Assessment, Second Edition*)
         f. Current medications
         g. Immunization history
         h. Review of systems
      2. Menstrual history
      3. Sexual history
      4. Elimination patterns
      5. Social history (see Box 20.3, *Advanced Pediatric Assessment, Second Edition*)

II. **Physical Examination**
    A. **Inspection of the Genitalia**
    B. **Palpation of the Genitalia**
    C. **Pelvic and Bimanual Exam**

SAMPLE DOCUMENTATION: MALE GENITOURINARY ASSESSMENT

Patient Name _____ Date of Birth_____ Date_____
Gender_____

I. **Health History**
   A. **Reason for Seeking Health Care** (e.g., routine well-child examination; genitourinary complaint [see Box 20.1, *Advanced Pediatric Assessment, Second Edition*])
      1. Past medical history
         a. Prenatal, birth, neonatal histories
         b. Congenital anomalies affecting the genitourinary tract

      c. Past hospitalizations (e.g., genitourinary injuries or infections)
      d. Surgical history
      e. Family medical history (see Box 20.2, *Advanced Pediatric Assessment, Second Edition*)
      f. Current medications
      g. Immunization history
      h. Review of systems
   2. Sexual history
   3. Elimination patterns
   4. Social history (see Box 20.3, *Advanced Pediatric Assessment, Second Edition*)

II. **Physical Examination**
   A. **Inspection of the Penis and Scrotum**
   B. **Palpation of the Penis and Scrotum**

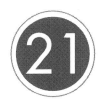

Assessment of the Musculoskeletal System

CHAPTER OVERVIEW

This chapter helps the learner to understand and refine the skills needed to perform an accurate age- and developmentally appropriate examination of the musculoskeletal system, to recognize deviations from normal, and to accurately record assessment findings.

Expected Learning Outcomes

After reading Chiocca, *Advanced Pediatric Assessment, Second Edition*, Chapter 21, the learner will be able to:

1. Obtain a thorough and accurate pediatric musculoskeletal history
2. Examine the musculoskeletal system in an age- and developmentally appropriate way
3. Analyze historical and physical assessment findings related to the musculoskeletal system and use these data to make accurate assessments and diagnoses
4. Accurately record history and physical assessment findings related to assessment of the musculoskeletal system

Essential Terminology

Abduction—movement away from the midline

Adduction—movement toward the midline

Circumduction—rotation or circular movements of the limbs

Diaphysis—the long shaft of a long bone

Dorsiflexion—movement of hands or feet upward

Epiphysis—rounded end of a long bone

Eversion—movement of an extremity or part of an extremity away from the body

Extension—increase in the angle of a joint; opposite of flexion

External rotation—turning of the anterior surface of a limb outward or away from the midline

Flexion—decrease in the angle of a joint; the opposite of extension

Genu valgum—the appearance of knock-knees seen in children beginning at 2 to 3 years and resolving by approximately 7 to 8 years; a normal variation

Genu varum—normal physiologic bowing of the legs in infants and toddlers

Growth plate (physis)—the portion of a long bone that is made of cartilage; does not fully ossify until early adulthood; injury to the growth plate can cause limb deformity, shortening of the bone, and arrest of growth

Hyperextension—increase in the angle of a joint beyond the normal angle

Internal rotation—turning of the anterior surface of a limb inward or toward the midline

Inversion—movement of an extremity or part of an extremity toward the body

Kyphosis—concave curvature of the thoracic spine

Lordosis—convex curvature of the spine; a normal variation in infants and toddlers

Luxation—dislocation

Metaphysis—the portion of the bone that lies between the epiphysis and diaphysis; the part of the bone that grows during childhood

Metatarsus adductus—the positional incurving of one or both feet caused by intrauterine positioning

Pes planus (flat foot)—a congenital condition of the foot involving laxity of the ligaments supporting the foot's longitudinal arch, causing flattening of the foot arch

Plantarflexion—movement of hands or feet downward

Pronation—turning of the palmar surface downward or toward the posterior surface of the body

Rotation—movement around a central axis

Scoliosis—lateral curvature of the spine

Subluxation—partial dislocation

Supination—turning of the palmar surface upward or toward the anterior surface of the body

Talipes equinovarus—true clubfoot, involving muscles, tendons, and bone

Valgus—deviation away from the midline

Varus—deviation toward the midline

Label the anatomic structures as indicated on these illustrations.

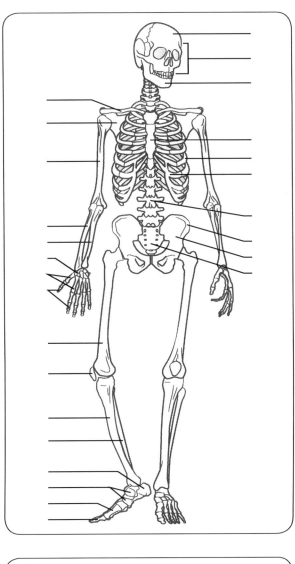

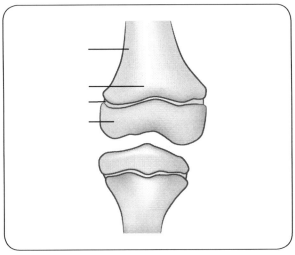

CRITICAL THINKING EXERCISES

Short-Answer Critical Thinking Exercises

1. Fill in the following box with the age-appropriate musculoskeletal assessment that should be conducted during the health supervision visit.

AGE	ASSESSMENTS
0–6 months	
6–12 months	
1–2 years	
2–3 years	
3–5 years	
5–12 years	
12 years and older	

2. Name some concerning musculoskeletal findings that may be found during the pediatric health supervision examination
3. What is the "growth plate" in the long bones of children? Why is any epiphyseal fracture of great concern if it occurs in a child?
4. Name some musculoskeletal complications of childhood obesity
5. In a child with fever, joint pain, and limp, what diagnostic tests would you order? What are your differential diagnoses?
6. Discuss why the developmental history is especially important when conducting the musculoskeletal assessment in children
7. Discuss fractures in children. Why are fractures less common in children than in adults? Why must the type and location of any fracture be fully evaluated in reference to the child's age and developmental level?

Critical Thinking Case Study Exercises

Exercise 1

Kimmie is a 3-year-old girl whose mother brings her to the clinic because Kimmie's right arm hurts and she is holding it still. Upon questioning, Kimmie's mother states that they were crossing the street that morning, and Kimmie attempted to dart out to meet a friend. At that point, her mother firmly grabbed her arm so Kimmie would not run in front of a car.

1. What other historical questions would you ask?
2. What physical examination would you do to further assess Kimmie's arm?
3. What condition do you suspect?

Exercise 2

Mia is a 6-month-old infant. Her prenatal, perinatal, and neonatal histories are unremarkable. Her current weight, length, and head circumference are all on the 75th percentile of the National Center for Health Statistics (NHCS) growth charts. Mia has a history of one afebrile upper respiratory infection at age 5 months. During her health maintenance examination, you notice that on her left thigh, she appears to have an extra gluteal fold.

1. What assessments should be made next?
2. Should the hips be assessed one at a time or simultaneously?
3. Is there anything in this infant's history that is relevant?
4. Should any other historical data be gathered?
5. What assessment findings would warrant an orthopedic referral?

Exercise 3

Amal is a 15-year-old boy who is brought to the urgent care center by his father. Amal is complaining of acute pain in the left hip. Currently, he cannot walk, and is holding his left leg in external rotation as he lies on the exam table. Current vital signs are: temperature 97.7°F (36.5°C); heart rate 124 bpm; respirations 20; blood pressure 130/90. His father reports that Amal's height is 68 inches; weight is 196 pounds.

1. Should any other historical data be gathered?
2. What specific questions should be asked?
3. What other physical assessments should be made?
4. What condition do you suspect? What is the next step?

Exercise 4

During the examination of a 2-day-old infant, you inspect foot position and alignment. You note that both feet are positioned in adduction. Both feet are flexible and can be abducted beyond the midline.

1. Is there anything in the prenatal or neonatal history that is essential to know?
2. Is this finding normal or abnormal?
3. Should the infant be referred to orthopedics?
4. What information should be given to the parents?

REVIEW QUESTIONS

1. Which of the following terms defines movement away from the midline?

   a. Abduction
   b. Adduction
   c. Flexion
   d. Extension

2. Physical findings associated with talipes equinovarus are:

   a. Medial deviation of the forefoot that is flexible and can be abducted beyond the midline
   b. Laxity of ligaments supporting the foot's longitudinal arch, causing the feet to be positioned in abduction

   c. Internal rotation of the foot with forefoot adduction involving muscles, tendons, and bone

   d. Marked inward deviation of the hand and an extremely short forearm

3. Assessment findings in an infant with developmental dysplasia of the hip can include:

   a. Negative Ortolani sign
   b. Positive Galeazzi sign
   c. Positive Trendelenburg sign
   d. Negative Barlow sign

4. Sustained clonus beyond six to eight beats, or clonus that continues past the neonatal period may indicate:

   a. Cerebral palsy
   b. Increased intracranial pressure
   c. Talipes equinovarus
   d. Dystonia

5. Which of the following assessment findings is within normal limits for the child's age?

   a. A toddler with lordosis
   b. A 3-year-old with genu varum
   c. A 12-year-old with genu valgum
   d. A 2-day-old with syndactyly

6. An antalgic gait indicates:

   a. Pain
   b. Infection
   c. Clubfoot
   d. Developmental dysplasia of the hip

7. A visible lateral curvature of the spine when the child is standing indicates:

   a. Lordosis
   b. Spina bifida
   c. Kyphosis
   d. Scoliosis

8. Assessment of the hips to detect developmental dysplasia of the hip is done at every well-child exam until age:

   a. 6 months
   b. 1 year
   c. 18 months
   d. 2 years

9. Tibial torsion can be caused by:

   a. Birth injury
   b. Trauma

    c. Viral illness

    d. Sickle cell disease

10. A 15-month-old boy is in the clinic for a well-child visit. You note increased muscle tone. This is a red flag for:

    a. Adam syndrome

    b. Cerebral palsy

    c. Down syndrome

    d. Muscular dystrophy

11. Until approximately what age is slight genu valgum (knock-knee) within normal limits?

    a. 7 to 8 years

    b. 8 to 9 years

    c. 9 to 10 years

    d. 10 to 11 years

12. A child who exhibits a positive Gower sign likely has a:

    a. Fracture

    b. Myopathy

    c. Hip infection

    d. Seizure disorder

13. Uneven knee height with knees flexed in a supine infant indicates:

    a. Genu varum

    b. Tibial torsion

    c. Developmental dysplasia of the hip

    d. Metatarsus adductus

14. A rapid and rhythmic, jerking movement of the foot caused by the sudden stretching of a tendon is termed:

    a. Tremor

    b. Clonus

    c. Nystagmus

    d. Myoclonus

15. Muscle strength in the lower extremities can be assessed in a 6-month-old infant by:

    a. Pulling the infant from the sitting to the standing position

    b. Placing the infant prone and observing whether the infant can crawl

    c. Performing the Ortolani maneuver

    d. Observing the infant try to pull to stand

16. The most common presenting symptom of neuromuscular disease in children is:

    a. Fatigue

    b. Muscle weakness

    c. Myoclonus
    d. Tremors

17. Genu varum ("bowlegs") is normal until age:

    a. 3 to 4 years
    b. 4 to 5 years
    c. 5 to 6 years
    d. 6 to 7 years

18. The varus deformity of both tibias caused by chronic obesity is:

    a. Osgood-Schlatter disease
    b. McMurray disease
    c. Blount's disease
    d. Werdnig-Hoffman disease

19. A marked limp or refusal to walk accompanied by fever, point tenderness, or limited range of motion in the hip suggests:

    a. Juvenile rheumatoid arthritis
    b. Osteomyelitis
    c. Cerebral palsy
    d. Sacroiliac inflammation

20. The forward bending test is an essential screening tool for:

    a. Lordosis in preschool children
    b. Kyphosis in school-aged children
    c. Torticollis in all age groups
    d. Scoliosis in school-aged children and adolescents

SAMPLE DOCUMENTATION: MUSCULOSKELETAL ASSESSMENT

Patient Name _____ Date of Birth _____ Date_____
Gender_____

I. **Health History**
   A. **Reason for Seeking Health Care** (e.g., routine well-child examination; musculoskeletal complaint)
      1. Past medical history
         a. Prenatal, birth, neonatal histories (skeletal deformities, syndromes)
         b. Chronic musculoskeletal conditions (e.g., juvenile rheumatoid arthritis)
         c. Past hospitalizations related to musculoskeletal system (e.g., injuries or infections)
         d. Injuries (fractures, dislocations, subluxations, sprains, strains)
         e. Surgical history
         f. Family medical history (e.g., genetic or idiopathic short stature; sickle cell disease)

g. Current medications

h. Social history (neglect [increased injuries], nutrition [obesity])

i. Review of systems

2. Developmental history (motor milestones)

3. Nutritional history (e.g., obesity, slipped capital femoral epiphysis)

4. Elimination patterns

II. **Physical Examination**

A. **Assessment of General Appearance**

B. **Inspection of Skin**

C. **Head, Neck, and Clavicles** (inspection and palpation)

D. **Gait**

E. **Upper Extremities and Shoulders** (inspection and palpation)

F. **Spine**

G. **Hips**

H. **Lower Extremities, Feet, and Ankles**

I. **Muscle Tone**

J. **Muscle Strength and Size**

K. **Involuntary Movements**

ASSESSMENT OF THE MUSCULOSKELETAL SYSTEM: WRITE-UP

Use the space provided here to document all subjective and objective findings using the SOAP rubric.

Subjective—(historical information; chief complaint; history of present illness)

_____

_____

Objective—(vital signs, physical examination findings, results of laboratory and other diagnostic tests)

_____

_____

Assessment—(diagnosis [use ICD-10 codes]; other health issues that are identified)

_____

_____

Plan—(treatment, medications, therapies, teaching, referrals, follow-up care)

_____

_____

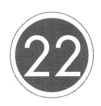

Assessment of the Neurologic System

CHAPTER OVERVIEW

This chapter helps to solidify the skills needed to perform an age- and developmentally appropriate neurologic history and examination of a pediatric patient, to recognize when the developmental examination is a necessary addition to the neurologic assessment, and to accurately record assessment findings.

Expected Learning Outcomes

After reading Chiocca, *Advanced Pediatric Assessment, Second Edition*, Chapter 22, the learner will be able to:

1. Obtain a thorough and accurate neurologic history for all pediatric age groups
2. Obtain a focused neurologic history of an ill or injured pediatric patient
3. Perform an age- and developmentally appropriate neurologic examination
4. Record all history and physical examination findings thoroughly and accurately

Essential Terminology

Amnesia—loss of memory

Aphasia—loss of expressive or receptive language abilities, or both; can occur in both spoken and written language

Apraxia—inability to perform purposeful movements in the absence of neurologic disease

Astereogenesis—inability to identify a familiar object through tactile recognition

Ataxia—muscle incoordination during voluntary movements

Athetosis—slow, involuntary writhing muscle movements; often seen in cerebral palsy

Chorea—abrupt, involuntary, jerky muscular movements

Clonus—repeated, involuntary rhythmic muscular spasms in response to sudden stretching

Decerebrate posturing—rigid extension of the extremities, with the toes pointed downward, and the head and neck arched backward; caused by brainstem lesions

Decorticate posturing—rigid flexion of the arms, with the fists clenched and held tightly on the chest, and the legs extended; caused by lesions of the corticospinal tract

Dysdiadochokinesia—inability to perform rapid alternating movements

Dysgraphesthesia—inability to recognize numbers or letters traced on the skin

Flaccidity—loss of muscle tone

Graphesthesia—the ability to identify shapes traced on the skin

Hypertonia—increased muscle tone

Hypotonia—decreased resistance to passive movement

Incoordination—low-level motor skills in the absence of neurologic disease

Mirror movements—simultaneous, contralateral, involuntary, identical movement that accompanies intentional movement

Motor—the portion of the neurologic examination that involves testing muscle movements

Myoclonus—rapid, sudden, jerking movement of a muscle or group of muscles

Nuchal rigidity—impaired neck flexion and stiffness in the cervical area due to muscle spasm of the extensor muscles of the neck; most often caused by meningeal irritation

Nystagmus—lateral oscillation of the eyes

Opisthotonos—severe arching of the back caused by injury or meningeal irritation

Papilledema—optic disc swelling caused by increased intracranial pressure

Paresthesia—a sensation of numbness or tingling anywhere on the body; can have multiple etiologies

Photophobia—severe sensitivity to light; may be associated with headache and nausea

Point localization—the ability to state exactly where the skin has been touched

Primitive reflexes—automatic, stereotypic reflexes that originate in the brainstem; with cortical maturity, primitive reflexes disappear

Proprioception—the body's ability to sense joint movement and position

Scissor gait—a gait abnormality often associated with cerebral palsy; characterized by leg muscle hypertonicity, lower extremity adduction, knee flexion, internal rotation of the hip, and plantarflexion of the ankle

Sensory—the portion of the neurologic examination that involves examination of the senses

Spasticity—stiff, rigid muscles with hyperactivity of deep tendon reflexes

Stereognosis—the ability to recognize objects by touch

Sunset sign—a manifestation of increased intracranial pressure that causes the sclera to be visible between the upper eyelid and iris

Superficial reflex—a motor response to stimulation of the skin

Tic—a habitual, repetitive muscular movement or vocalization

Two-point discrimination—the ability to discriminate simultaneous touch at two different points on the skin

CRITICAL THINKING EXERCISES

Short-Answer Critical Thinking Exercises

1. Name the structures of the central nervous system (CNS).
2. What are the major functions of the following parts of the cerebral cortex?

   a. Frontal lobe
   b. Parietal lobe
   c. Temporal lobe
   d. Wernicke's area
   e. Broca's area

3. What is the blood–brain barrier and what is its function? What are some clinical implications of the functions of the blood–brain barrier?
4. What is the spinal cord and what is its function? Discuss the ascending and descending tracts.
5. What is the peripheral nervous system (PNS)? How does it differ from the CNS? What structures comprise the PNS and what are their functions?
6. Name the 12 cranial nerves. For each cranial nerve, state whether the nerve's function is sensory, motor, or mixed, and how its function is tested in children of various ages.
7. What are some anatomic and physiologic differences in the CNS and PNS in infants and children?
8. Why are the prenatal, perinatal, and neonatal histories important and relevant to the neurologic assessment, especially for children aged 3 years and younger?
9. Discuss the pediatric neurologic health history and its components.
10. What parts of the neurologic examination can be done just by observing the infant or child?
11. Why is the developmental assessment relevant to the neurologic assessment in infants and children?
12. Discuss the following components of the neurologic assessment for each pediatric age group:

    a. Mental status examination
    b. Cranial nerve assessment
    c. Assessment of cerebellar function
    d. Proprioception
    e. Pain
    f. Reflex testing

13. What neurologic assessments should be made when an infant or child has an acute neurologic injury or infection? Be specific. Do the assessments differ based on age? Why?

Critical Thinking Case Study Exercises

Exercise 1

Kaitlin is a 6-year-old girl who presents to the urgent care center accompanied by her parents. Kaitlin is being held in her father's lap, and has clearly been crying. Approximately 1 hour ago, Kaitlin was riding a two-wheeled bicycle, when she lost control and fell off the bicycle onto a concrete sidewalk. Her parents have brought her in for care because they are concerned that Kaitlin is becoming drowsy, but they are not sure if it is because of the fall, or simply due to the fact that she had an unusually late bedtime the night before. Her current vital signs are: temperature 98.4°F (36.9°C); pulse 96 bpm; respirations 24; blood pressure 92/60.

1. What other parts of Kaitlin's injury history should be obtained?
2. What, if anything, is important to know about Kaitlin's past medical history?
3. What questions should be asked as part of the focused history?
4. What specific neurologic assessments should be obtained?
5. What, if any, laboratory or imaging assessments are important?

Exercise 2

Michael, aged 6 months, was born at 31 weeks gestation. He was intubated and ventilated with supplemental oxygen for the first 3 weeks of his life. Michael was discharged from the neonatal intensive care unit at corrected age 38 weeks. Michael is at the clinic for immunizations and a well-child examination.

1. In reviewing Michael's past medical history what is it important to know about the following:

   a. Prenatal history
   b. Perinatal history
   c. Neonatal history

2. How will Michael's past medical history affect what the provider expects to see on his physical examination?
3. What specific neurologic assessments should be obtained for Michael?
4. What physical findings are to be expected, given Michael's history?
5. What specific developmental assessments should be considered for Michael?
6. Should Michael have attained developmental milestones for a 6-month-old infant? Why or why not?

Exercise 3

Natasha is a 5-year-old girl in need of a kindergarten physical. She has not had a well-child examination for 3 years and does not attend preschool. Her developmental assessment reveals an alert, playful, friendly child with expressive speech and fine motor delays. She does not recognize colors and cannot copy shapes or write her name.

1. What questions should be asked regarding Natasha's past medical history?
2. What information is it important to gather about Natasha's social history?
3. What information is it important to gather about Natasha's developmental history?
4. What specific neurodevelopmental assessments should be performed on Natasha?

Exercise 4

Maura, aged 16 years, presents to the health care provider accompanied by her mother, with complaints of chronic headaches.

1. What is it important to know about Maura's past medical history?
2. What is it important to know about Maura's social history?
3. What information should be obtained as part of the history of present illness?
4. What should be included in Maura's physical examination?

REVIEW QUESTIONS

1. The most sensitive indicator of a child's neurologic status is:

   a. Mood and affect
   b. Gait and balance
   c. Cranial nerve assessment
   d. Level of consciousness

2. Which of the following assessments indicates potential cerebellar dysfunction?

   a. Ataxia
   b. Graphesthesia
   c. Hearing deficits
   d. Stereognosis

3. To assess vestibular function of the acoustic nerve in a child, the examiner would:

   a. Perform the whisper test
   b. Perform the Romberg test
   c. Perform the Weber test
   d. Perform the Rinne test

4. To examine for the function of the hypoglossal nerve in a child, the examiner would:

   a. Ask the child to identify tastes
   b. Ask the child to stick out his or her tongue
   c. Test the child's ability to swallow
   d. Ask the child to nod his or her head from side to side

5. Which of the following is the most appropriate method of evaluating cerebellar function in a preschool-aged child?

   a. Perform the Romberg test
   b. Cranial nerve examination
   c. Observation of heel-to-toe walking
   d. Ask the child to perform the finger-to-nose test

6. Injury to Wernicke's area of the cerebral cortex results in:

   a. Executive function deficits
   b. Expressive aphasia
   c. Receptive aphasia
   d. Memory loss

7. The presence of Brudzinski's sign indicates:

   a. Increased intracranial pressure
   b. Meningeal irritation
   c. Cerebellar dysfunction
   d. Spinal cord injury

8. A 3-year-old child suffered a severe traumatic brain injury. The examiner would expect this child's Babinski reflex to be:

   a. Negative
   b. Positive
   c. Fluctuating, depending on intracranial pressure
   d. Unable to be assessed

9. A 5-year-old boy is new to the clinical practice and presents for a kindergarten physical. During the exam, his gait is assessed. No limp or ataxia is noted, but he is toe-walking. The provider asks his parents if this is how he normally walks and they say yes. Which of the following parts of the child's past medical history are important to assess?

   a. Previous history of hyperactive deep tendon reflexes
   b. Previous history of lower extremity injury
   c. History of perinatal or neonatal hypoxia or asphyxia
   d. History of high fevers in infancy

10. Which of the following developmental assessment findings requires an in-depth neurologic assessment?

    a. Delayed expressive language milestone achievement
    b. Poor school performance
    c. Loss of developmental skills
    d. Poor social skills with peers

11. Which of the following assessment findings indicates increased intracranial pressure?

    a. Papilledema on fundoscopic examination
    b. Nuchal rigidity

    c. Numbness and tingling

    d. Hyperactive deep tendon reflexes

12. A normal response to the elicitation of the Achilles tendon reflex is:

    a. Flexion of the toes

    b. Plantarflexion

    c. Extension of the great toe with fanning of the remaining toes

    d. Extension of the toes

13. To test the sensory function of the trigeminal nerve in an infant, the examiner would:

    a. Elicit the startle reflex

    b. Elicit the gag reflex

    c. Assess direct and consensual papillary response to light

    d. Elicit the corneal (blink) reflex

14. To elicit the plantar reflex:

    a. Ask the child to slide the heel of the foot along the opposite shin

    b. Place a vibrating tuning fork on the child's ankle and ask the child when the vibration stops

    c. Strike the lateral aspect of the sole of the foot with the end of the reflex hammer

    d. Ask the child to perform a heel-to-toe walk

15. A child has been hit by a car while riding her bicycle. The Glasgow Coma Scale assessment reveals a total score of 10. This is considered indicative of a:

    a. Mild head injury

    b. Moderate head injury

    c. Severe head injury

    d. Normal finding

16. Which of the following postural reflexes should disappear by age 12 to 24 months?

    a. Positive support

    b. Landau

    c. Parachute

    d. Protective extension sitting position

17. The Glasgow Coma Scale includes all of the following assessment areas *except*:

    a. Eye opening

    b. Thought processes

    c. Motor response

    d. Verbal response

18. Because of the need for the child's cooperation during assessment, the sensory examination is not typically conducted until age:

    a. 2 years
    b. 3 years
    c. 4 years
    d. 5 years

19. Neurologic soft signs, when found on neurologic examination, indicate:

    a. A likely history of severe asphyxia and a poor neurologic outcome
    b. A sign of a moderate cerebral ischemic injury and likely motor and cognitive delays
    c. A minor abnormality and often resolve by late school age to adolescence
    d. A lingering effect of traumatic brain injury

20. Which of the following neurologic assessments tests proprioception?

    a. Assessment of the child's ability to identify direction of movement
    b. Assessment of pain
    c. Assessment of the child's ability to identify hot and cold temperature
    d. Assessment of ability to hop in place

SAMPLE DOCUMENTATION: NEUROLOGIC ASSESSMENT

Patient Name_____ Date of Birth_____ Date_____
Gender_____

I. **Health History**
   A. **Reason for Seeking Health Care** (e.g., routine well-child examination; neurologic complaint)
      1. Past medical history
         a. Prenatal, birth, neonatal histories
         b. Chronic health conditions (e.g., epilepsy, migraines)
         c. Past hospitalizations (e.g., meningitis)
         d. Injuries (e.g., traumatic brain injury)
         e. Surgical history (e.g., craniotomy)
         f. Family medical history (e.g., congenital hypothyroidism)
         g. Current medications
         h. Immunization history
         i. Review of systems
      2. Neurologic history (see *Advanced Pediatric Assessment, Second Edition*, Chapter 22, for age-specific assessment questions)
      3. Developmental history
      4. Social history

II. **Physical Examination**
    A. **Vital Signs**
    B. **Mental Status Evaluation**
    C. **Cranial Nerve Assessment**
    D. **Motor Assessment**
    E. **Assessment of Cerebellar Function**

    F. Sensory Examination
    G. Reflex Testing
        1. Use scale to quantify responses, 0 to 4+
        2. Test reflexes bilaterally
    H. Pain
    I. Developmental Assessment

NEUROLOGIC ASSESSMENT: WRITE-UP

Use the space provided here to document all subjective and objective findings using the SOAP rubric.

Subjective—(historical information; chief complaint; history of present illness)

_____

_____

Objective—(vital signs, physical examination findings, results of laboratory and other diagnostic tests)

_____

_____

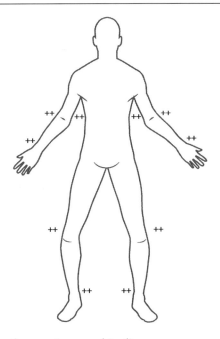

Record results of reflex testing on this diagram.

Assessment—(diagnosis [use ICD-10 codes]; other health issues that are identified)

_____

_____

Plan—(treatment, medications, therapies, teaching, referrals, follow-up care)

_____

_____

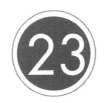

Assessment of Mental Disorders in Children and Adolescents

CHAPTER OVERVIEW

This chapter helps the pediatric health care provider to become more adept in the assessment of mental health in infants, children, and adolescents. The pediatric health care provider will become familiar with common pediatric mental health conditions, age-appropriate assessments and diagnoses, and common pediatric mental health screening tools.

Expected Learning Outcomes

After reading Chiocca, *Advanced Pediatric Assessment, Second Edition*, Chapter 23, the learner will be able to:

1. Identify common mental health problems in children and adolescents
2. Discuss the prevalence and common co-morbidities of selected pediatric mental health disorders
3. Identify and use common mental health screening assessment tools for children and adolescents
4. Perform an age-appropriate mental status examination on a child and adolescent
5. Identify and discuss the categories of historical mental health assessment data for children and adolescents
6. Recognize the signs and symptoms of mental illnesses in children and adolescents that signal an immediate safety threat to self or others
7. Demonstrate the ability to record all health assessment findings accurately and completely

Essential Terminology

Addiction—the compulsive physiologic and psychological dependence on a behavior or a habit-forming substance

Affect—observable expression of feeling or emotion

Behavior—the manner in which one acts in a particular situation; affected by family, peer group, socioeconomic status, and culture; may also be affected by diet, medication, and physiologic or psychological illness

Mood—a temporary feeling or state of mind

Phobia—a persistent, developmentally abnormal, irrational fear resulting in a compulsion to avoid what is feared

Temperament—individual personality characteristics and behaviors

CRITICAL THINKING EXERCISES

Short-Answer Critical Thinking Exercises

1. Discuss the effect of temperament on a child's or adolescent's mental health.
2. Discuss how a child's or an adolescent's social situation can affect his or her mental health.
3. Discuss the signs of grief and loss in each age group. What are some common causes of grief in children?
4. Name the screening tools commonly used to assess for attention deficit hyperactivity disorder, autism, anxiety disorders, and depression.
5. Compare and contrast normal versus pathologic separation anxiety.
6. Compare and contrast normal fears versus phobias. In what age group are fears most prevalent and considered developmentally appropriate?
7. Compare and contrast tantrums and stubbornness with oppositional defiant disorder.
8. What are some risk factors for and co-morbidities related to self-mutilation in adolescent girls?
9. How does anorexia nervosa affect each body system? What are some physical signs of anorexia nervosa that may be observed in the primary care setting?
10. Discuss the various types of mood disorders in children and adolescents. What are some presenting signs and symptoms that can be observed in the primary care setting?
11. What is the difference between a neat, organized, or highly motivated child and one who has obsessive-compulsive disorder?
12. Explain why all young children and adolescents should be screened for suicidality during the primary care visit.
13. Why is mental health assessment essential in every pediatric health care visit?

Critical Thinking Case Study Exercises

Exercise 1

Mia is a 5-year-old girl who lives in a high crime area. Several instances of gun violence have occurred in the past 6 months. Three months ago, while walking to a convenience store, Mia, along with her mother, father, and 6-year-old brother, witnessed a shooting. The shooting victim was in clear view, and the gunman pushed past Mia's father as he ran away, knocking him over. Today, Mia is at the clinic for her well-child visit, accompanied by both parents. They say they are concerned because Mia has started "acting like a baby," sucking her thumb, wetting the bed, saying her stomach hurts, and insisting on sleeping with her parents. Mia's parents state that their son "acted like a baby" when they first brought Mia home from the hospital "to get attention"; but they do not know why she is acting like this. Mia's brother has not shown similar behavior in recent weeks, which makes Mia's parents even more concerned that "she needs medication."

1. What other, more specific, historical questions should the provider ask the parents?
2. What should the provider ask about Mia's social history?
3. What should the provider ask about Mia's medical history?
4. Is Mia's behavior within normal limits for age and developmental level? Why or why not?
5. What, if any, screening tools should be used to assess Mia's behavior?

Exercise 2

David is a 15-year-old male teen who presents for his annual physical. When the provider asks if there are any issues or concerns, David's mother states that he is irritable all the time, has occasional angry outbursts, and recently has begun spending more time alone in his room and less time with his friends. She also states that she has noticed that David is staying up later, and is difficult to awaken for school. When asked, both David and his mother admit that his grades have gone from As and Bs to mainly Ds.

1. When obtaining the social history, what are the important questions to ask?
2. When obtaining the family history, what are the important questions to ask?
3. What, if anything, in David's medical history is important to know?
4. What other information about David's recent behavior should be obtained from his mother?
5. The provider asks David's mother to step out of the room. What questions should David be asked when alone?
6. What screening tool(s) or self-report questionnaire(s) would be useful in this scenario?
7. When conducting David's physical examination, what should the provider focus on?
8. What is the single most important question to ask in this health care encounter?

Exercise 3

Aaron is a 5-year-old boy who presents to the clinic 1 month after his kindergarten physical. His mother states that he has not been able to attended a full day of school because he screams, cries, and clings when she drops him off. When the teacher tells his mother to just leave and allow Aaron to adjust, she is called approximately 1 hour later to pick him up because he is still crying and panicked about being separated from his mother. Further questioning reveals that Aaron did not attend preschool, wakes up frequently with nightmares, and has had recurrent abdominal pain.

1. What other parts of Aaron's past medical history are important to know?
2. When obtaining the social history, what are the important questions to ask?
3. When obtaining the family history, what are the important questions to ask?
4. What part of Aaron's the developmental history is relevant in this scenario?
5. Is Aaron's behavior within normal limits, given his age and social history?
6. Is there any objective screening tool that could be used in this scenario?

Exercise 4

Lisa is a 17-year-old who presents to the school-based health center with complaints of a sore throat and "feeling hot." During the physical examination, the nurse practitioner notices several cuts on Lisa's forearms in various stages of healing. The nurse practitioner asks Lisa directly if she has ever cut or hurt her skin on purpose, and she says yes.

1. What follow-up questions should be asked?
2. What is the most important follow-up question to ask?
3. What communication techniques (see Chapter 3) can the nurse practitioner use to ensure that Lisa feels safe in disclosing information?
4. What parts of Lisa's social history are important to know?
5. What parts of Lisa's medical history are important to know?
6. Discuss the issue of confidentiality as it relates to adolescent self-injury. What should the nurse practitioner tell Lisa about ensuring confidentiality?
7. What are some common risk factors for adolescent self-injury?
8. What are some psychiatric co-morbidities that may accompany adolescent self-injury?
9. What other physical assessments should be made to assess for these co-morbidities?
10. How should the nurse practitioner follow up with Lisa?

REVIEW QUESTIONS

1. A mental health assessment is being conducted on 16-year-old Melissa. Which of the following statements should *not* be kept confidential?

   a. "I have been sexually active with three boys."
   b. "I sometimes smoke pot."
   c. "I sometimes drink wine from my parent's alcohol cabinet."
   d. "Sometimes I feel like ending my life."

2. Which of the following somatic complaints often accompanies anxiety disorders in children?

   a. Headache
   b. Somnolence

c. Bradycardia
d. Seizures

3. Which of the following assessment findings is indicative of anxiety that is outside normal limits?

a. A 15-month-old who cries intensely when she sees her mother gather her car keys and purse
b. A 4-year-old who is afraid to take a bath because he is afraid of being sucked down the drain
c. An 8-year-old who wakes up nightly, seeking parental reassurance regarding fears and concerns about what will happen the next day
d. An adolescent who is worried and preoccupied about social acceptance and social competence at school

4. During a health maintenance visit, the mother of an 8-year-old boy says that he has received several warnings at school regarding his behavior. His teacher and the school social worker have documented that he loses his temper easily, repeatedly defies the teacher and school rules, argues with adults at school, and deliberately annoys his classmates. The health care provider should do a full screening for:

a. Social phobias
b. Depression
c. Attention deficit hyperactivity disorder
d. Oppositional defiant disorder

5. Signs of nonsuicidal self-injury may include all of the following *except*:

a. Emaciated appearance
b. Wearing long-sleeved clothing in warm weather
c. Overt suicidal ideation
d. Scarring on visible skin

6. Common fears among school-aged children include:

a. Loud noises
b. Separation
c. Peer rejection
d. Physical well-being

7. Somatic indicators of anxiety in children may include:

a. Nightmares
b. Abdominal complaints
c. Irritability
d. Shaking

8. The mother of an 11-year-old boy is concerned because he has recently begun refusing to go to school, his teachers state that he seems extremely nervous when asked to speak in class, and he refuses invitations to school

events or parties. Based on this information, the health care provider suspects:

a. Social phobia
b. Panic disorder
c. Selective mutism
d. Conduct disorder

9. Which of the following signs in a 13-year-old girl raises suspicion for bulimia nervosa?

a. Lanugo
b. Dull hair
c. Hypertension
d. Enlarged parotid glands

10. The hallmark of obsessive-compulsive disorder is:

a. Fear
b. Worry
c. Impulsivity
d. Repetition

11. When conducting an overall screening for cognitive, emotional, and behavioral disorders in children aged 11 years and older, a suggested screening tool is:

a. SAD PERSONS Scale
b. Modified Checklist for Autism in Toddlers (M-CHAT)
c. *DSM-5*-based diagnostic criteria
d. Pediatric Symptom Checklist

12. Signs of anorexia nervosa may include:

a. Amenorrhea
b. Hypertension
c. Tachycardia
d. 90% of expected weight

13. The parents of a 6-year-old child bring him to the clinic with concerns about his behavior. The parents have received numerous notes from his teacher and school social worker regarding his inability to stay in his seat during class, his failure to pay attention to the teacher, frequent class interruptions, and forgetting to bring completed assignments to class. The child has no cognitive delays, nor has he demonstrated any oppositional behavior. The provider should screen this child for:

a. Anxiety disorder
b. Autistic spectrum disorders
c. Attention deficit hyperactivity disorder
d. Oppositional defiant disorder

14. Which of the following events in a 6-year-old child's life would prompt screening for posttraumatic stress disorder (PTSD)?

    a. Change of schools twice in the past year
    b. Death of the family pet
    c. Family dislocation due to a hurricane
    d. Loss of a beloved security object

15. The most important component to the diagnosis of depression in children and adolescents is:

    a. The physical examination
    b. The clinical interview
    c. Results of self-report questionnaires
    d. Assessment of co-morbid psychiatric disorders

16. A school-aged child displays a pattern of behavior that includes bullying, excessive teasing of the family dog, deliberate destruction of siblings' toys, and excessive lying. This child is displaying signs of:

    a. Conduct disorder
    b. Oppositional defiant disorder
    c. Sociopathy
    d. Bipolar disorder

17. The likelihood of suicidality increases with:

    a. Obesity
    b. Social phobia
    c. Attention deficit hyperactivity disorder
    d. Mood disorders

18. The assessment finding of high concern for acute suicide risk in a highly depressed teen is:

    a. Low self-esteem
    b. Active hallucinations
    c. Excessive sleep
    d. History of substance abuse

19. Adolescents with bipolar disorder are at risk for all of the following *except*:

    a. Suicide
    b. Sexually transmitted infections
    c. Self-mutilation
    d. Sleep disturbances

20. A 9-year-old child of political refugees has recently arrived from a country that has been war-torn for 10 years. This child requires a school physical.

During the health encounter, this child should also be screened for all of the following *except*:

a. PTSD
b. Depression
c. Anxiety and panic disorder
d. Obesity

SAMPLE DOCUMENTATION: ASSESSMENT OF MENTAL HEALTH

Patient Name _____ Date of Birth _____ Date _____
Gender_____

I. **Health History**
   A. **Reason for Seeking Health Care**
   B. **Past Medical History**
      1. Prenatal, birth, neonatal histories (e.g., prematurity, prolonged ventilation, extracorporeal membrane oxygenation)
      2. Injuries (type and severity, mechanism of injury)
      3. Emergency room visits (dates and reason for visit)
      4. Chronic conditions
      5. Past hospitalizations
      6. Surgical history
      7. Family medical history
      8. Current medications
         a. Prescription
         b. Over the counter
         c. Include exact dose, frequency, time of last dose given, reason for medication
      9. Alternative therapies used
      10. Immunization status (note delays)
      11. Review of systems
   C. **Nutritional History**
      1. Meal schedule
      2. 24-hour food recall for past 3 to 5 days
      3. Bottle propping
      4. Appetite
      5. Voracious appetite
      6. Vomiting/rumination
      7. Dental visits
   D. **Developmental History**
      1. Milestones reached
      2. Behavior
      3. Temperament
      4. Prolonged screen time
   E. **Sleep History**
      1. Hours per day
      2. Difficulty sleeping/insomnia/hypersomnia
      3. Nightmares

F. Social History
1. Maternal support systems
2. Family stresses/crises
3. Parental mental illness or addiction
4. Poor parental bonding
5. Inappropriate dress for weather
6. Teenage parents
7. Parental knowledge deficits
8. Poverty/homelessness
9. School performance
10. Behavior at school
11. Truancy
12. Frequent school tardiness

II. **History of Present Illness (Mental Health Complaint)**

III. **Physical Examination**
A. **Vital Signs**
B. **Anthropometric Measurements**
1. Weight
2. Length/height
3. Head circumference (age 3 years and younger)
4. Weight for length/height (both height and weight below fifth percentile occur with longstanding neglect)
5. Body mass index (age 2 years and older)
6. Plot all measurements on growth charts
C. **Mental Status Exam**
D. **Behavioral Assessment for Age**
1. Mood
2. Affect
3. Behavior
4. Parent–child interaction
5. Eye contact
6. Smiling/interaction
7. Presence/absence of stranger anxiety (infants/toddlers)
8. Anxiety
9. Agitation
10. Apathy
11. Dislike of being touched/held
12. Preference for inanimate objects over toys or social interaction
13. Irritability
14. Lethargy
E. **Developmental Assessment**
1. Objective developmental assessment for age (use formal developmental assessment tool)
2. Temperament

    F. **Skin Assessment**
1. Hygiene
2. Scars on knuckles (Russell's sign)
3. Sores around cheeks or mouth

    G. **Neurologic Assessment**

    H. **Nutritional Assessment**
1. Tooth decay
2. Skin turgor
3. Note emaciated or malnourished appearance
4. Overweight/obesity
5. Alteration in elimination patterns

MENTAL HEALTH ASSESSMENT: WRITE-UP

Use the space provided here to document all subjective and objective findings using the SOAP rubric.

Subjective—(historical information; chief complaint; medical and psychiatric co-morbidities)

_____

_____

Objective—(vital signs, physical examination findings, results of laboratory and other diagnostic tests; results of screening instruments)

_____

_____

Assessment—(diagnosis [use ICD-10 codes]; other health issues that are identified)

_____

_____

Plan—(treatment, medications, therapies, teaching, referrals, follow-up care)

_____

_____

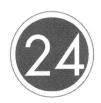

Assessment of Child Abuse and Neglect

CHAPTER OVERVIEW

One of the most critical assessments the pediatric health care provider can make is to determine whether a child is being neglected or abused. The health care provider must have sharp assessment skills to be able to recognize the various types of child neglect, differentiate between intentional and unintentional injuries, identify the subtle signs of emotional or verbal abuse, and sensitively gather subjective and objective data when sexual abuse is suspected.

Expected Learning Outcomes

After reading Chiocca, *Advanced Pediatric Assessment, Second Edition*, Chapter 24, the learner will be able to:

1. Discuss the characteristics of the parent, child, and environment that increase the risk for child abuse or neglect
2. Describe the elements of the pediatric history and physical examination that may indicate abuse or neglect
3. Discuss the special importance of the health history in cases of suspected child abuse or neglect
4. Demonstrate the ability to differentiate between intentional and unintentional injuries in infants and children
5. Explain the importance of obtaining an accurate, nonbiased, and complete history and physical examination when any type of child abuse or neglect is suspected
6. Compare and contrast cutaneous findings seen in children who have had traditional methods of healing used versus inflicted, intentional injuries
7. Demonstrate the ability to record all health assessment findings accurately and completely

Essential Terminology

Child abandonment—the most extreme form of child neglect; involves the parent or guardian abandoning a child outside the parameters of safe relinquishment provided by law

Coin rubbing ("cao gio")—a traditional Southeast Asian method of healing involving vigorous rubbing of a coin on the chest to treat fever, cough, and congestion; may be confused with physical abuse

Corporal punishment—the use of physical force to control a child's behavior

Cupping—a traditional Southeast Asian method of healing used to treat respiratory complaints; involves placing a glass cup on the child's chest, lighting a candle, and holding the flame at the base of the cup in order to create suction; this leaves a circular area of ecchymosis and petechiae that may be mistaken for abuse

Educational neglect—failure to ensure that a child attends school each day or adheres to any special education needs set forth by the teacher or school district

Emotional abuse—a pattern of behavior directed at a child by a parent or caregiver that aims to belittle, berate, humiliate, or criticize

Emotional neglect—failure of the parent or caregiver to meet the child's emotional needs

Medical neglect—failure to obtain necessary medical care for a child

Moxibustion—a type of acupuncture that involves burning; may be confused with physical abuse due to small burns left on skin after treatment

Munchausen syndrome by proxy (MSP)—a condition in which an adult perpetrator (most often the mother) directly causes or lies about an illness in a child in order to gain attention and sympathy for herself or himself; most often perpetrated on children age 6 years and younger

Neglect—acts of omission in caring for a child, such as deprivation of life's basic necessities including clean and safe housing, provision of adequate types and amounts of nutritious food, basic hygiene, weather-appropriate clothing, education, and emotional support

Physical abuse—the nonaccidental injury of a child by a parent, sibling, relative, or caregiver

Sexual abuse—the act of a forcing a child to engage in sexual activity; the perpetrator is known to the child

Supervisory neglect—parental or caregiver failure to provide age-appropriate supervision to infants or young children

Verbal abuse—the deliberate attempt on the part of an adult to harm a child with words; includes but is not limited to belittling, insulting, berating, humiliating, blaming, criticizing, mocking, or shaming

CRITICAL THINKING EXERCISES

Short-Answer Critical Thinking Exercises

1. What is the most common type of child maltreatment in the United States?
2. What are some parent or caregiver risk factors for abuse or neglect of children?

3. What are some characteristics of children that place them at increased risk for abuse?
4. Name some environmental stressors that increase risk for child abuse and neglect.
5. Discuss the difference between verbal and emotional abuse of children.
6. What are some examples of red flags for abuse or neglect that can present during the routine health maintenance examination?
7. What injury sites on a child's body raise suspicion for child abuse?
8. Discuss how the health care provider can differentiate intentional and unintentional burns in an infant or a young child.
9. At what age should a child begin to be asked about his or her own injuries or suspected abuse? How should the provider phrase the questions? Discuss developmental variations when obtaining the history from a child or adolescent who may have been abused or neglected.
10. Why is skeletal trauma in children younger than age 2 years likely the result of intentional injury? What specific type of fracture is particularly suspicious for intentional injury of a preambulatory child?
11. Name some pattern injuries and common items used to inflict these types of injuries.
12. What types of caregiver discipline practices increase risk for emotional and physical abuse of the child?
13. What are some injuries or illnesses that are often mistaken for abuse or neglect in children?
14. What are some traditional healing methods that may mimic physical abuse?
15. Discuss some important factors to consider when obtaining the history in a case of suspected child abuse or neglect.
16. What is the most important criterion to consider when making the decision to report a child's injury to child protective services?
17. Discuss some physical and behavioral indicators of child sexual abuse.
18. What are some conditions of the anogenital region that may mimic child sexual abuse?
19. Why is objective, accurate documentation so crucially important with suspected child abuse and neglect?

Critical Thinking Case Study Exercises

Exercise 1

Angela is a 12-month-old White infant girl who is brought to the clinic for a health maintenance examination. Hospital records indicate that she was born at 37 weeks gestation without complications. Her birth weight was 3.18 kg (7 pounds) (25%); birth length 19.5 inches (49.5 cm) (25%); and head circumference 13.5 inches (34.3 cm) (25%). The newborn screen was negative. Angela has not received any health care since birth; her mother says "she hasn't been sick." Angela is bottle fed, and her mother gives her whole milk, approximately 16 to 24 ounces per day, on no particular feeding schedule. Her mother cannot be sure exactly how much milk Angela consumes, because she props the bottle and some of the milk leaks out of the top of the bottle. Angela's mother gives her table food such as pasta, mashed potatoes, and fast food, but her mother says she spits it out. Her other solid food consumption is mainly dry cereal and applesauce. Administration of the Ages and Stages Questionnaire (ASQ) reveals global delays.

Angela's weight today is 6.4 kg (14 pounds) (<3%); length is 26 inches (66 cm) (<3%); and head circumference is 16.5 inches (41.9 cm) (<3%). Angela's vital signs are within normal limits for age. On physical examination, Angela is small and disinterested in her surroundings. She does not cry when the health care provider takes her from her mother's lap and places her on the exam table. Physical findings include loose skin folds, severe diaper rash, and overall poor hygiene. Cardiac rate and rhythm are normal and no murmur is heard. Breath sounds are clear bilaterally. Her physical examination is otherwise unremarkable.

Angela's developmental assessment reveals good head control; she does not pull to stand or cruise. She does not attempt to pick up small objects and is only mildly interested in toys and social games such as peek-a-boo. With direct interaction, Angela does not smile, coo, or vocalize but she does turn to sound. After crying briefly, Angela sucks on her tongue to comfort herself.

1. What other historical data must be obtained?
2. What aspects of Angela's family or social history should the provider be sure to obtain?
3. What other details must be gathered about Angela's nutritional history?
4. In addition to the information given above, what should Angela's physical examination include?
5. Are Angela's growth parameters within normal limits?
6. Is Angela's behavior age appropriate?
7. Discuss Angela's developmental assessment.
8. What is the difference between organic and nonorganic failure to thrive?
9. What laboratory tests, if any, should be ordered for Angela?
10. Should Angela receive her age-appropriate immunizations today?
11. What, if any, referrals should be made?

Exercise 2

A 15-month-old Hispanic boy presents to the clinic for an episodic visit accompanied by both parents. The chief complaint includes runny nose, fever, diarrhea, and vomiting for 3 days. The physical examination reveals a mildly dehydrated but otherwise healthy toddler. During the physical examination, bruising in various stages of healing is noted over the abdomen just under the umbilicus. When asked about the bruising, the parents state that they put a belt on their son's pants so he does not remove them while they are in the process of toilet training him, and they think this may have left a mark. Further inspection by the examiner reveals a circular, macular, bluish-purple lesion just above his sacrum. The parents deny that their son has had any history of abnormal bleeding or bruising. All lab studies are normal.

1. Does the history that the parents give for the abdominal bruising match the type and degree of injury?
2. Are the bruises on this child's abdomen more likely intentional or unintentional? Why or why not?
3. Is the lesion on this child's sacrum suspicious for abuse? Why or why not?
4. Is this child at risk for physical abuse? Why or why not?
5. What should the next step be for this child?

Exercise 3

The parents of a 13-month-old boy have brought him to the emergency room (ER) stating that he accidentally scalded himself with hot water when he pulled a pot from the top of the stove. Upon inspection, the child's anterior chest reveals a fresh first- to second-degree burn, centered in the sternal area, moving down toward the umbilicus in a tapering pattern. As the burn gets further from the anterior chest, its edge becomes irregular. No other injuries are noted on the child and he appears well-nourished and developmentally within normal limits.

1. Does the history that the parents give for this child's burn match the type and degree of injury?
2. Should this child's parents be interviewed separately?
3. Is this burn likely intentional or unintentional? Explain.
4. Is this child at risk for physical abuse? If so, why?
5. What should the recommended course of action be for this child?

Exercise 4

Tam is a 3-year-old Asian boy who was brought to the ER with a 4-day history of fever, runny nose, productive cough, and ear pain. Tam's physical examination reveals copious nasal drainage, a fever of 101.2°F (38.4°C), crackles on the right side, and an erythematous, bulging tympanic membrane on the right. While auscultating Tam's lungs, the health care provider notes circular bruising and burns on his posterior chest.

1. What is the first question the heath care provider should ask about these bruises and burns?
2. What other historical questions must be asked in this case?
3. What parts of Tam's past medical history are relevant in order to make a correct diagnosis?
4. Should Tam and his parents be interviewed separately or together?
5. What should Tam's physical examination focus on?
6. What diagnostic studies, if any, are necessary?
7. What is the differential diagnosis for this child?

Exercise 5

Susannah, aged 4 years, is brought to the clinic by her mother because of persistent vaginal discharge. Her mother is clearly uncomfortable discussing the chief complaint with the health care provider. Susannah's mother is vague about the onset of the vaginal discharge, but does mention that Susannah has had a history of poor personal hygiene after both urination and defecation. When asked which family members live in the home, Susannah's mother states that currently she and Susannah live at home but that a boyfriend (not Susannah's father) had been living with them until a month ago, when she asked him to move out. When the health care provider asks Susannah's mother why she asked her boyfriend to leave, and she begins to cry.

1. What other historical questions must be asked in this case?
2. What parts of Susannah's past medical history are relevant in order to make a correct diagnosis?

3. Should Susannah and her mother be interviewed separately or together?
4. What should the physical examination focus on?
5. What diagnostic studies, if any, are necessary?
6. What is the differential diagnosis for this child?
7. What, if any, referrals should be made?

Exercise 6

Bree is an 18-month-old girl who has been brought to the ER by her mother with complaints of intractable crying. Bree's mother is unsure about exactly when the crying started but thinks it may have been 2 to 3 days ago when Bree fell off a chair at home. The mother states that, at first, Bree cried "very hard," but then seemed fine. She denies that Bree is having any difficulties eating or sleeping and denies any changes in Bree's elimination patterns. Currently, Bree is afebrile, her heart rate is 140 bpm and regular, respirations are 20, and blood pressure is 110/66. She is crying inconsolably. Bree's physical examination is unremarkable except that while she is crying in her mother's lap, she is kicking and the left leg is moving but her right leg is not.

Bree's mother's boyfriend arrives in the ER approximately 1 hour later, while Bree and her mother are in the radiology department. He introduces himself and asks for Bree and her mother, stating that Bree is "the baby who fell off the swing at the park." When Bree and her mother return from the radiology department, and the radiologist informs the health care provider that Bree has a spiral fracture of the right femur.

1. What other parts of the medical and psychosocial history are important to obtain?
2. When obtaining this history, should Bree's mother and her boyfriend be interviewed separately or together?
3. Should Bree be interviewed separately?
4. Are there any parts of the history presented here that raise red flags for abuse?
5. Given the finding of a spiral fracture of the right femur what should the physical examination focus on?
6. What diagnostic studies, if any, are necessary?
7. Are there any red flags or risk factors for abuse in Bree's history and physical examination?
8. What should the next step be in caring for Bree?

REVIEW QUESTIONS

1. Which of the following statements is *not* correct regarding potentially abusive families?

   a. Teenage mothers are less likely to release frustration by striking out at their child
   b. Abusive parents have difficulty controlling their anger
   c. Domestic violence often occurs in families that physically abuse their children
   d. Abusive families are often more socially isolated and have fewer support systems

2. Which of the following is a true statement?

   a. Intentional burns tend to be asymmetrical, irregular, partial thickness, and reflective of the child's motor abilities
   b. Spiral and metaphyseal chip fractures in children carry a low index of suspicion for abuse
   c. Before reporting suspected inflicted injuries to a child, the health care provider must be able to prove an infant or child has been abused
   d. Bruises over bony prominences such as the extensor surfaces of the lower leg, knee, elbows, and forehead are the most common sites of accidental bruising

3. Which of the following characteristics of infants and young children places them at high risk for abuse?

   a. Prolonged weaning time
   b. Extended bedtime rituals
   c. Crying and toilet training
   d. Early achievement of expressive language

4. A 2-year-old child is brought to the clinic after falling off a slide at the park and sustaining three small bruises to the face. All of the following components of the health history should raise suspicion of child abuse *except*:

   a. The parents seek medical assistance immediately after the injury
   b. The type and degree of injury is incompatible with the history
   c. The parents delay seeking medical attention for the injury
   d. The parents give different histories when asked to describe what happened

5. Which of the following is a red flag for nonorganic failure to thrive in a 12-month-old?

   a. Clinging to the primary caregiver during the physical examination
   b. No stranger anxiety
   c. Weight-for-age at the 10th percentile on growth chart
   d. Weight-for-length at the 10th percentile on growth chart

6. Which of the following assessments of a child's family and social history can indicate an increased risk for child abuse?

   a. Maternal depression
   b. The parent leaves the children with a babysitter or family member several afternoons a week
   c. The parents attend parenting classes
   d. The mother's primary support system is several women in the area with children of similar ages

7. An inflicted immersion burn is characterized by:

   a. A tapering distribution
   b. A clear line of demarcation
   c. An inverted triangle shape
   d. A splash pattern

8. All of the following are risk factors for child abuse or neglect *except*:

   a. Being an only child
   b. Parental substance abuse
   c. Exposure to domestic violence
   d. Child has history of being a premature infant

9. The health care provider suspects physical abuse of a 6-year-old girl with an injured leg and interviews her separately from her parents. Which of the following is an example of an appropriate question to ask this child?

   a. "Did your mom's boyfriend hurt you?"
   b. "Did your mom do that to you?"
   c. "What happened to your leg?"
   d. "Does your mom ever hit you?"

10. Indicators of emotional abuse may include:

    a. Immunization delays
    b. Depressed affect
    c. Poor dental health
    d. Unexplained injuries

11. All of the following, reported by the parents during the interview, are red flags for child abuse *except*:

    a. Blaming the incident on a sibling
    b. Delay in seeking care
    c. No clear explanation for the injury
    d. Parents adamantly stick to their story

12. When taking an interval history for a 2-year-old toddler, the pediatric health care provider notes four ER visits in the past year for treatment of injuries. This may indicate all of the following *except*:

    a. Physical abuse
    b. Neglect
    c. Developmental delay
    d. Malnutrition

13. Which type of intentional injuries to a child often present with nonspecific signs such as irritability, fatigue, or poor appetite?

    a. Central nervous system injuries
    b. Musculoskeletal trauma
    c. Eye injuries
    d. Oral injuries

14. Children younger than 4 years of age are more susceptible to shaken baby syndrome because of all of the following characteristics *except*:

    a. Proportionately larger head
    b. Friable intracranial vasculature

   c. Weak neck muscles

   d. Weaker muscle tone

15. Indicators of child sexual abuse may include all of the following *except*:

   a. Retinal hemorrhages

   b. Encopresis

   c. Phobias

   d. Enuresis

16. Intentional cigarette burns are typically:

   a. On older children

   b. Of superficial depth

   c. Partial thickness

   d. In areas that are concealed by clothing

17. Which of the following conditions may be confused with intentional burns?

   a. Idiopathic thrombocytopenic purpura

   b. Impetigo

   c. Erythema multiforme

   d. Henoch-Schönlein purpura

18. A mother brings her 7-year-old boy into the clinic to be examined after he made a statement to her that his uncle was touching his private parts. Brief inspection of the anogenital region reveals three small wart-like lesions. In order to make a correct differential diagnosis, the examiner must examine this child's anogenital region more closely. What position should be used to perform the exam?

   a. Supine or left side-lying

   b. Right side-lying

   c. Knee-chest position

   d. Prone

19. A 30-month-old boy is in the office for his annual health maintenance examination. The pediatric health care provider notes anal fissures, perianal skin tags, and some other flesh-colored pedunculated lesions. His mother denies that the child has any history of constipation, but does recall seeing blood in his diaper on a few occasions. His health history is otherwise unremarkable. The social history reveals that the child has no siblings, the child's biological father is not involved, and the child's mother has had several live-in male partners. In order to ensure a correct diagnosis, what should the health care provider do next?

   a. Nothing; these are normal findings

   b. Ask for the contact information for the mother's partners and interview them

   c. Contact a board-certified sexual assault nurse examiner (SANE) to interview the mother, examine the child further, and collect evidence

   d. Call the police; this represents sexual abuse

20. Signs of shaken baby syndrome may include all of the following *except*:
    a. Extensive bruising of the head
    b. Subdural hematoma
    c. Intracranial edema
    d. Retinal hemorrhages

SAMPLE DOCUMENTATION: CHILD ABUSE AND NEGLECT

Careful documentation of suspected child abuse or neglect is very important. Medical terminology may be misinterpreted by child protective services or law enforcement officials, with potentially tragic results. All documentation must be clear, without medical jargon or abbreviations, and completely objective. A body diagram should be used to indicate the locations of any visible injuries. Any statements made by the child, parent, caregiver, family member, friend, or sibling must be charted verbatim and in quotation marks.

Sample Documentation: Suspected Child Neglect

Patient Name _____ Date of Birth _____ Date _____
Gender_____

I. **Health History**
   A. **Reason for Seeking Health Care**
   B. **Past Medical History**
      1. Prenatal, birth, neonatal histories (e.g., prematurity, prolonged ventilation, extracorporeal membrane oxygenation)
      2. Injuries (type and severity, mechanism of injury)
      3. ER visits (dates and reason for visit)
      4. Chronic conditions
         a. Congenital heart disease
         b. Chronic respiratory diseases (e.g., cystic fibrosis, bronchopulmonary dysplasia)
         c. Cleft lip/palate
         d. Gastroesophageal reflux disease
         e. Malabsorption syndromes
         f. Endocrine dysfunction
         g. AIDS
      5. Hospitalizations
      6. Surgical history
      7. Family medical history
      8. Medications taken
         a. Prescription
         b. Over the counter
         c. Include exact dose, frequency, time of last dose given, reason for medication
      9. Alternative therapies used
      10. Immunization status (note delays)
      11. Review of systems

C. **Nutritional History**
  1. Meal schedule
  2. 24-hour food recall for last 3 to 5 days
  3. Bottle propping
  4. Refusing solids
  5. Anorexia
  6. Voracious appetite
  7. Vomiting/rumination
  8. Dental visits
D. **Developmental History**
  1. Milestones reached
  2. Behavior
  3. Temperament
  4. Prolonged screen time
E. **Sleep History**
  1. Hours per day
  2. Difficulty sleeping/insomnia/hypersomnia
  3. Nightmares
F. **Social History**
  1. Maternal support systems
  2. Family stresses/crises
  3. Parental mental illness or addiction
  4. Poor parental bonding
  5. Inappropriate dress for weather
  6. Teenage parents
  7. Parental knowledge deficits
  8. Poverty/homelessness
  9. School performance
  10. Truancy
  11. Frequent school tardiness

II. **Physical Examination**
  A. **Vital Signs**
  B. **Anthropometric Measurements**
    1. Weight
    2. Length/height
    3. Head circumference (age 3 years and younger)
    4. Weight for length/height (both height and weight below fifth percentile occur with longstanding neglect)
    5. Body mass index (age 2 years and older)
    6. Plot all measurements on growth charts
  C. **Behavioral Assessment for Age**
    1. Parent–child interaction
    2. Eye contact
    3. Smiling/interaction
    4. Presence/absence of stranger anxiety (infants/toddlers)
    5. Apathy
    6. Dislike of being touched/held

      7. Preference for inanimate objects over toys or social interaction

      8. Irritability

      9. Lethargy

  D. **Developmental Assessment**

      1. Objective developmental assessment for age (use formal developmental assessment tool)

      2. Temperament

  E. **Skin Assessment**

      1. Hygiene

      2. Rashes

      3. Infections

  F. **Nutritional Assessment**

      1. Skin turgor

      2. Note emaciated or malnourished appearance

Suspected Child Neglect: Write-Up

Use the space provided here to document all subjective and objective findings using the SOAP rubric.

Subjective—(historical information; chief complaint; history of present illness)

_____

_____

Objective—(vital signs, physical examination findings, results of laboratory and other diagnostic tests)

_____

_____

Assessment—(diagnosis [use ICD-10 codes]; other health issues that are identified)

_____

_____

Plan—(treatment, medications, therapies, teaching, referrals, follow-up care)

_____

_____

Sample Documentation: Suspected Child Physical Abuse

Patient Name _____ Date of Birth _____ Date _____
Gender _____

  I. **Health History**

    A. **Reason for Seeking Health Care**

    B. **History of Injury**

      1. How, when, and where injury occurred

      2. Who was with child when he or she was injured?

3. Other witnesses to injury
4. Ask child how injury occurred (age appropriate) with parent out of room

C. Past Medical History
1. Injuries (type and severity, mechanism of injury)
2. ER visits (date and reason for visit)
3. Chronic conditions
   a. Bleeding disorders
   b. Osteogenesis imperfecta
   c. Connective tissue disorders
   d. Metabolic diseases
4. Hospitalizations
5. Surgical history
6. Family medical history
7. Medications taken
   a. Prescription
   b. Over the counter
   c. Include exact dose, frequency, time of last dose given, reason for medication
8. Alternative therapies used
9. Immunization status
10. Review of systems
11. Social history

II. Physical Examination
A. Vital Signs
1. Temperature
2. Heart rate
3. Respiratory rate
4. Blood pressure

B. Anthropometric Measurements
1. Weight
2. Length/height
3. Head circumference (age 3 years and younger)
4. Weight for length (age 2 years and younger)
5. Body mass index (age 2 years and older)
6. Plot all measurements on growth charts

C. Behavioral Assessment for Age
1. Irritability
2. Lethargy

D. Parent–Child Interaction
1. Does child look to parent(s) when crying or frightened?
2. Child withdrawn/submissive/clingy with parent(s)?
3. Do parents react to child's needs?
4. Do parents show an appropriate degree of concern?
5. Child's behavior without parent(s) present

E. Parental Behavior
1. Assess parent's history of any injuries assessed
2. Is history compatible with the type/degree of injury?

    3. Is the parent's version of the history of the child's injury vague?

    4. Does the history change?

    5. Do the parents give different histories?

    6. Is there a significant delay between the time of injury and time when medical care was sought?

F. **Developmental Assessment**

    1. Normal for age

    2. Delayed

    3. Global or delays noted or in one or developmental domains

G. **Skin Assessment**

    1. Bruises (note location, color)

    2. Abrasions

    3. Lacerations

    4. Burns (note location, depth, stage of healing)

    5. Pattern injuries

    6. Restraint/tourniquet marks

    7. Bite marks

    8. Oral injuries (e.g., torn frenulum)

    9. Scars/old injuries

H. **Abdominal Assessment**

    1. Presence of bruises

    2. Irritability

    3. Vomiting

    4. Lethargy

    5. Abdominal distention

    6. Signs of shock

I. **Musculoskeletal Assessment**

    1. Range of motion

    2. Pain

    3. Muscle tone

    4. Bruising

    5. Visible or palpable deformities of extremities

J. **Neurologic Assessment**

    1. Level of consciousness (lethargy, irritability)

    2. Behavior

    3. Reflexes

    4. Respiratory changes

    5. Cranial nerve assessment

    6. Presence of retinal hemorrhages

    7. Poor feeding

    8. Vomiting

    9. Seizures

    10. Fractures

Suspected Child Physical Abuse: Write-Up

Use the space provided here to document all subjective and objective findings using the SOAP rubric.

Subjective—(historical information; chief complaint; history of present illness)

_____

_____

Objective—(vital signs, physical examination findings, results of laboratory and other diagnostic tests)

_____

_____

Document physical findings of injuries on a body map.

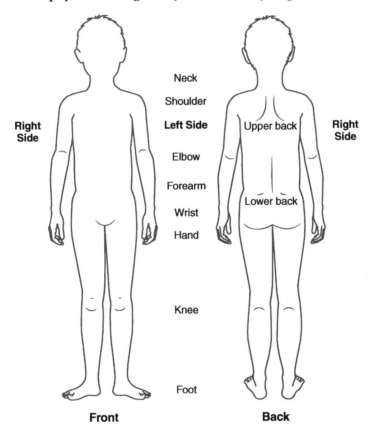

Neck
Shoulder
Left Side   Upper back
Elbow
Forearm
Lower back
Wrist
Hand

Knee

Foot

Right Side

Right Side

Front

Back

Assessment—(diagnosis [use ICD-10 codes]; other health issues that are identified)

_____

_____

Plan—(treatment, medications, therapies, teaching, referrals, follow-up care)

_____

_____

Sample Documentation: Suspected Child Sexual Abuse

Patient Name _____ Date of Birth _____ Date _____
Gender_____

I. Health History
  A. Reason for Visit
  B. History of Present Illness (e.g., burning on urination, discharge, enuresis)
   1. Obtain history from child separate from parents (age 3 years and older) that is brief and gathers enough data to confirm suspicion of sexual abuse
   2. Forensic interview at child advocacy center
  C. Past Medical History
   1. Anogenital history
      a. Anogenital injuries (e.g., playground, bicycle injuries)
      b. Pain
      c. Bleeding
      d. Discharge
      e. Recurrent urinary tract infections
      f. Labial adhesions
      g. Vulvovaginitis
   2. Age of menarche
   3. Last menstrual period
   4. Mental health
      a. Depression
      b. Suicidal ideation
      c. Attention deficit hyperactivity disorder
      d. Substance abuse
      e. Posttraumatic stress disorder
      f. Phobias
   5. Recurrent abdominal pain
   6. Enuresis
   7. Encopresis
  D. Social History
   1. Change in child's behavior
      a. Acting out
      b. Fear of being around perpetrator
      c. Expression of sexual knowledge inappropriate for age
      d. Sexualized behaviors
      e. New fears or phobias
      f. New development of eating disorders
      g. Depression
      h. Suicide attempts
      i. Any witnesses to sexual abuse
   2. School performance
      a. New onset of poor school performance
      b. School refusal
  E. Sleep History
   1. Insomnia

2. Hypersomnia
3. New-onset nightmares
4. Nocturnal enuresis

II. **Physical Examination**
  A. **Behavioral Assessment**
    1. Disclosure made by child during visit
    2. Withdrawn
    3. Clingy to parent
  B. **Head-to-Toe Physical Examination to Assess for Injuries**
    1. Bruises
    2. Abrasions
    3. Lacerations
  C. **Anogenital Assessment** (note: findings may be normal despite the occurrence of sexual abuse)
    1. Girls
      a. Inspection
        i. Sexual maturity rating
        ii. Vagina
          (a) Hymenal injuries (tears/lacerations)
          (b) Erythema
          (c) Bruising
          (d) Edema
          (e) Bleeding
          (f) Discharge
          (g) Lesions (e.g., warts, herpetic lesions)
        iii. Anus
          (a) Erythema
          (b) Bruising
          (c) Tears/lacerations
          (d) Bleeding
          (e) Dilation
          (f) Lesions (e.g., warts, herpetic lesions)
          (g) Discharge
      b. Palpation
        i. Avoid palpation of prepubertal hymen (sensitive to pain)
        ii. Use cotton-tipped swab to palpate pubertal hymen
      c. Signs of pregnancy
    2. **Boys**
      a. Inspection
        i. Sexual maturity rating
        ii. Descension of testes
        iii. Penis
          (a) Lesions
          (b) Rashes
          (c) Discharge
        iv. Anus
          (a) Erythema
          (b) Bruising
          (c) Tears/lacerations

      (d) Abrasions
      (e) Edema
      (f) Bleeding
      (g) Dilation
      (h) Lesions (e.g., warts, herpetic lesions)
      (i) Discharge
      (j) Perianal scarring
    b. Palpation of testes (masses)

Suspected Child Sexual Abuse: Write-Up

Use the space provided here to document all subjective and objective findings using the SOAP rubric.

Subjective—(historical information; chief complaint; history of present illness)

_____

_____

Objective—(vital signs, physical examination findings, results of laboratory and other diagnostic tests)

_____

_____

Assessment—(diagnosis [use ICD-10 codes]; other health issues that are identified)

_____

_____

Plan—(treatment, medications, therapies, teaching, referrals, follow-up care)

_____

_____

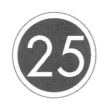

The Complete History and Physical Examination: From Start to Finish

CHAPTER OVERVIEW

This chapter helps the learner to pull together the assessments of all the individual body systems into one complete physical examination, tailoring the approach to the assessment to the child's age and developmental stage.

Expected Learning Outcomes

After reading Chiocca, *Advanced Pediatric Assessment, Second Edition,* Chapter 25, the learner will be able to:

1. Demonstrate knowledge of the skills of inspection, palpation, auscultation, and percussion
2. Demonstrate correct use of physical examination equipment as appropriate for the child's age
3. Integrate and synthesize the knowledge gained from learning individual body systems assessments to conduct a complete, head-to-toe physical examination on a pediatric patient of any age
4. Conduct the complete pediatric physical examination in the correct sequence for age and developmental level
5. Know the developmental variations that may need to be employed when conducting a complete physical examination on a pediatric patient of any age
6. Accurately document findings

Essential Terminology

Anthropometric measurement—measurement of body weight, height (or length), head circumference

Developmental variation—changes in the approach to the physical examination according to age or developmental level

General appearance—an overall cursory evaluation of the child before commencing the actual physical examination

Sequencing—the order in which the physical examination takes place

CRITICAL THINKING EXERCISES

Short-Answer Critical Thinking Exercises

1. What is the recommended sequence of the complete physical examination for each age group?
2. Why does the recommended sequence of the complete physical examination vary among age groups?
3. Name some ways in which the provider could prepare children of different age groups for the physical examination.
4. What are some developmental considerations that affect the approach to the physical examination?
5. Name some variations in position and location of the physical examination in infants and toddlers that help to facilitate the exam.
6. For each body system, list the important areas to assess in each age group.

Critical Thinking Case Study Exercises

Exercise 1

Jenny and Jamie are 12-month-old twins who are at the clinic for their health maintenance examinations. They are accompanied by their mother, grandmother, and 5-year-old brother. Both twins are fussy and hungry, and their brother is asking you questions about everything you are doing during the visit.

1. Which twin should be examined first, or does it matter?
2. Where would you conduct the physical examination of each twin?
3. In what sequence would you conduct the physical examination?
4. Would you involve the mother, grandmother, or big brother? Why or why not? If yes, how would you do so?

Exercise 2

Cindy is an 18-month-old toddler who was initially very wary of you when you entered the examination room to conduct her physical exam. She cried and clung to her mother but is now intent on a cardboard picture book that you gave her. It is time to begin the physical exam.

1. What are some developmental considerations that should be kept in mind as you begin the physical exam?
2. What parts of the physical exam could you perform just by watching Cindy look at the book?
3. As you approach Cindy to start the exam, she puts the book down, starts to cry, and walks toward her mother, reaching her arms up to be held. What information can you glean from this that can be documented as part of Cindy's physical assessment?
4. List the steps you would take to complete Cindy's physical examination.

Exercise 3

Nick is a 14-year-old boy who has come to the clinic for a sports physical. He is very shy and appears uncomfortable discussing his health. When it comes time for the physical examination, he asks if he has to take his clothes off.

1. Should the sequence of Nick's physical examination be altered in any way? Why or why not?
2. What body system would you examine last? Is this an alteration of what you would plan to do even if Nick was not demonstrating discomfort?
3. What could the provider do to make Nick feel more at ease before the physical examination begins?

REVIEW QUESTIONS

1. The body mass index should be measured in all children beginning at age:

    a. 1 year
    b. 2 years
    c. 3 years
    d. 4 years

2. In a sleeping infant, which of the following assessments should be conducted *first*?

    a. Inspect tone and general appearance
    b. Gently palpate skin for temperature
    c. Palpate pedal pulses
    d. Auscultate lung and heart sounds

3. Which of the following children may be more cooperative and less fearful during the physical examination if allowed to touch and listen through the stethoscope?

    a. A crying 12-month-old
    b. A 2-year-old who is pushing you away during the otoscopic exam
    c. An adolescent who is curious and wants to delay the physical exam
    d. A preschooler who is asking why you have to listen to his lungs and if something is inside his chest

4. In the infant, which of the following systems is examined last?

    a. Genitalia
    b. Ears, nose, and throat
    c. Spine and extremities
    d. Chest and heart

5. In the adolescent, which of the following systems is examined last?

    a. Genitalia
    b. Ears, nose, and throat

c. Spine and extremities

d. Chest and heart

6. Part of your assignment as a nurse practitioner is to make rounds in the nursery two mornings a week. You are about to examine Pablo, a 2-day old with an unremarkable history, when he begins to cry vigorously. The appropriate next step is to:

a. Delay the exam until Pablo stops crying

b. Try to get him to stop crying by feeding him, then proceed with the exam

c. Take the opportunity to examine his oral cavity while he is crying, then try to console him so he quiets

d. Proceed with the physical examination as usual, beginning with the chest and heart

7. At what age should the child's standing height begin to be measured?

a. 1 year

b. 2 years

c. 3 years

d. 4 years

8. In which of the following age groups would you normally conduct a portion of the history and physical examination with the parent out of the room?

a. Toddlers—they cry more when they see their parent

b. Preschoolers—they like to show off in front of the parent by asking a lot of questions

c. School-aged children—they are more likely to talk about what they like to eat with their parent out of the room

d. Adolescents—they are less likely to give honest answers about drug or alcohol use, depression, or school problems with the parent present

9. Frida is a toddler who is very uncooperative during the physical examination. Which of the following can help you to conduct the exam?

a. Ask the mother or primary caregiver to step out of the room; this may be causing the crying

b. Ask the mother or primary caregiver to feed Frida; this may quiet her down

c. Ask Frida's mother to hold her on her lap and face you as you sit facing the mother, knee-to-knee, and examine Frida there

d. Give Frida a pacifier

10. In which age group can the provider begin to conduct the complete physical examination in a head-to-toe sequence?

a. Infants

b. Toddlers

c. Preschoolers

d. School-aged children

THE COMPLETE PHYSICAL EXAMINATION

Equipment and Supplies Necessary for the Physical Examination of Infants, Children, and Adolescents

For vital sign measurement:
- Thermometers (oral, axillary, rectal, tympanic)
- Pediatric stethoscope with bell and diaphragm
- Various infant and pediatric-sized blood pressure cuffs
- Sphygmomanometer
- Doppler

For anthropometric measurements:
- Beam balance scale to measure weight (both infant and adult platform scales)
- Paper to line infant scale
- Measuring board to measure recumbent length in infants (may also measure recumbent length on paper-covered surface)
- Wall-mounted stadiometer (for most accurate measurement of standing height)
- Paper or metal tape measure (to measure head or arm circumference)
- Skinfold calipers (e.g., Lange calipers) to measure skinfold thickness
- Age- and gender-specific Centers for Disease Control and Prevention growth charts
  - ❑ Weight-for-age (birth–36 months)
  - ❑ Length-for-age (birth–36 months)
  - ❑ Weight-for-length (birth–36 months)
  - ❑ Head circumference-for-age (birth–36 months)
  - ❑ Weight-for-age (2–20 years)
  - ❑ Stature-for-age (2–20 years)
  - ❑ Weight-for-stature (2–20 years)
  - ❑ Body mass index-for-age (2–20 years)

For integumentary assessment:
- Ruler with centimeter markings
- Wood's lamp
- Magnifying glass

For head and neck:
- Small glass of water (for child to swallow during thyroid gland assessment)
- Nasal specula

For ears:
- Otoscope with pneumatic bulb
- Ear curettes for cerumen removal
- Tuning fork

For eyes:
- Penlight
- Ophthalmoscope
- Snellen eye chart, "tumbling E" chart, and Allen cards for vision screening
- Cover card

(continued)

For nose and oral cavity:
- Penlight
- Tongue depressors
- Otoscope (to view inside nares)

For lungs, heart, and abdomen:
- Stethoscope with appropriately sized bell and diaphragm
- Doppler to assess peripheral pulses

For musculoskeletal exam:
- Measuring tape

For neurologic exam:
- Reflex hammer
- Tuning fork
- Tongue depressor
- Sharp and dull testing instruments
- Penlight (to test pupillary reflex)
- Cotton-tipped swabs (to test corneal and blink reflexes)
- Salt and sugar (to test discrimination of sweet and sour taste)
- Coffee, alcohol, or soap (to test smell)

For female genital exam:
- Gloves
- Vaginal specula (including pediatric sized)
- Lubricant
- Sterile cotton-tipped swabs or applicators
- Bifid spatula
- Saline
- Slides, fixative, and container
- Specimen containers

For developmental assessment:
- Selected developmental assessment tools (e.g., Ages and Stages; see *Advanced Pediatric Assessment, Second Edition*, Chapter 2)
- Puppets, small blocks (for assessing pincer grasp), stacking toys, and squeak toys (also for gaining infant's or toddler's attention and for assessing hearing)

Miscellaneous supplies:
- Pediatric history and physical forms
- Wristwatch or clock with a second hand
- Calculator (to calculate body mass index; drug doses)
- Variously sized paper gowns
- Examination drapes
- Paper to line examination table
- Variously sized syringes and needles
- Puncture-resistant sharps disposal container
- Paper towels and tissue
- Cotton balls
- Culture media
- Potassium hydroxide
- Gauze

SAMPLE DOCUMENTATION: NEONATE AND INFANT (BIRTH THROUGH 1 YEAR)

Patient Name _____ Date of Birth _____
Source of Information _____ Relationship to Patient (mother, father, grandparent, caregiver)

Subjective Data

I. History
   A. Prenatal History
   B. Neonatal History
      1. Apgar score
   C. Postnatal History
      1. Gestational age assessment
   D. Maternal History
      1. Age
      2. Gravida
      3. Para
      4. Past medical history
      5. Modality of conception
      6. Drug, alcohol, tobacco use while pregnant
II. Immunizations
   A. Allergies
   B. Past Medical History
   C. Past Surgical History
   D. Family Medical History
   E. Injuries/Ingestions
   F. Emergency Room Visits
   G. Current Medications
III. Nutrition
   A. Breast Milk
   B. Formula
   C. Solids, How Much, How Often
   D. Bottle Propping
IV. Elimination
   A. Number of Wet Diapers and Stools Per Day
   B. Character of Stools
V. Safety
   A. Back to Sleep
   B. Car Seat
   C. Water and Burn Safety
   D. Fall Prevention
   E. Choking Prevention
   F. Tobacco Smoke Exposure
   G. Smoke and Carbon Monoxide Detectors in Home
VI. Sleep
   A. Hours of Sleep
   B. Number of Naps
VII. Social
   A. Living Situation; Who Lives in Home
   B. Maternal Depression/Support System

VIII. **Developmental**
   A. **Gross Motor** (e.g., head control, sitting, pulling to stand, walking)
   B. **Fine Motor** (e.g., grasping)
   C. **Social** (e.g., smiling, interaction with toys)
   D. **Cognitive** (e.g., progress achieving object permanence)

Objective Data

Vital Signs

   1. Temp _____
   2. Apical heart rate _____
   3. Respiratory rate _____
   4. Blood pressure _____
   5. Weight _____kg_____pounds_____ounces
   6. Length _____cm_____inches
   7. Head circumference _____cm_____inches
   8. Parent–child interaction _____
   9. General appearance _____
  10. Skin _____
  11. Head _____
  12. Face _____
  13. Eyes _____
  14. Ears _____
  15. Nose _____
  16. Mouth/throat _____
  17. Neck _____
  18. Thorax and lungs _____
  19. Breast _____
  20. Heart _____
  21. Abdomen _____
  22. Upper extremities _____
  23. Lower extremities _____
  24. Neurologic/reflexes _____
  25. Genitalia _____
  26. Rectum/anus _____
  27. Developmental assessment _____
  28. Results of laboratory tests _____ (e.g., hemoglobin, hematocrit, lead, neonatal screening)

   Assessment:_____

   Plan:_____

SAMPLE DOCUMENTATION: TODDLER AND PRESCHOOLER (AGES 1–6 YEARS)

Patient Name _____ Date of Birth _____
Source of Information _____ Relationship to Child (mother, father, grandparent, caregiver)

Subjective Data

I. History
 A. Prenatal
 B. Neonatal
  1. Apgar score
 C. Postnatal
  1. Gestational age assessment
 D. Maternal
  1. Age
  2. Gravida
  3. Para
  4. Past medical history
  5. Modality of conception
  6. Drug, alcohol, tobacco use while pregnant
 E. Past Medical History
 F. Past Surgical History
 G. Family Medical History
 H. Immunizations
 I. Allergies
 J. Injuries/Ingestions
 K. Emergency Room Visits
 L. Current Medications
II. Nutrition
 A. Typical Meals, and Snacks
 B. Amount and Type of Milk Ingested Each Day
 C. Amount of Juice/Soft Drinks Consumed Each Day
 D. Amount of Physical Activity/Screen Time Per Day
III. Elimination
 A. Number of Wet Diapers and Stools Per Day
 B. Character of Stools
 C. Toilet Training Progress After Age 2 Years
IV. Safety
 A. Car Seat/Booster Seat
 B. Water and Burn Safety
 C. Fall Prevention
 D. Bicycle Helmet
 E. Choking Prevention
 F. Tobacco Smoke Exposure
 G. Smoke and Carbon Monoxide Detectors in Home
V. Sleep
 A. Length of Sleep
 B. Number of Naps
 C. Where Child Sleeps
 D. Night Terrors (preschoolers)
 E. Insomnia
 F. Excessive Sleeping
 G. Chronic Bedwetting After Toilet Training

VI. Social
- A. Living Situation; Who Lives in Home
- B. Maternal Depression/Support System

VII. Growth and Development
- A. Age at Which Child
  1. Held head up
  2. Rolled over front to back; back to front
  3. Sat unsupported
  4. Crawled
  5. Walked alone
  6. Said first word
  7. Said first sentences
  8. Toilet trained
  9. Dressed without help

VIII. Review of Systems
- A. General
- B. Integument
- C. Head
- D. Eyes
- E. Nose
- F. Ears
- G. Mouth
- H. Throat
- I. Neck
- J. Nodes
- K. Chest
- L. Respiratory
- M. Cardiovascular
- N. Gastrointestinal
- O. Genitourinary
- P. Gynecologic
- Q. Musculoskeletal
- R. Neurologic
- S. Endocrine
- T. Lymphatic

Objective Data

Vital Signs

1. Temp _____
2. Heart rate _____
3. Respiratory rate _____
4. Blood Pressure _____
5. Weight _____kg _____pounds_____ ounces
6. Length _____cm _____inches
7. Height (> age 2 years) _____cm _____inches
8. Body mass index (> age 2 years) _____
9. Head circumference _____cm _____inches
10. Parent–child interaction _____

General Appearance

1. Skin _____
2. Head _____
3. Face _____
4. Eyes _____
5. Ears _____
6. Nose _____
7. Mouth/throat _____
8. Neck _____
9. Thorax and lungs _____
10. Breast _____
11. Heart _____
12. Abdomen _____
13. Upper extremities _____
14. Lower extremities _____
15. Neurologic/reflexes _____
16. Genitalia _____
17. Rectum/anus _____
18. Developmental assessment _____
19. Results of laboratory tests _____ (e.g., hemoglobin, hematocrit, lead)

Assessment: _____

Plan: _____

SAMPLE DOCUMENTATION: SCHOOL-AGED CHILD (AGES 6–12 YEARS)

Patient Name _____ Date of Birth _____
Source of Information _____ Relationship to Child (mother, father, grandparent, caregiver)

Subjective Data

I. Past Medical History
II. Past Surgical History
III. Family Medical History
IV. Immunization History
V. Allergies
VI. Injuries/Ingestions
VII. Emergency Room Visits
VIII. Current Medications
IX. Nutrition
    A. Typical Meals and Snacks
    B. Amount of Juice/Soft Drinks/Junk Food Consumed Each Day
    C. Amount of Physical Activity/Screen Time Per Day
X. Elimination
    A. Constipation
    B. Diarrhea

    C. Enuresis
    D. Encopresis
  XI. Safety
    A. Bicycle Helmet
    B. Stranger Safety
    C. Seatbelts
    D. Smoke and Carbon Monoxide Detectors
    E. Street Safety
    F. Bullying
  XII. Sleep
    A. Hours of Sleep
    B. Bedtime
  XIII. Social
    A. Living Situation; Who Lives in Home
    B. Maternal Depression/Support System
  XIV. School Performance
  XV. Review of Systems
    A. General
    B. Integument
    C. Head
    D. Eyes
    E. Nose
    F. Ears
    G. Mouth
    H. Throat
    I. Neck
    J. Nodes
    K. Chest
    L. Respiratory
    M. Cardiovascular
    N. Gastrointestinal
    O. Genitourinary
    P. Gynecologic
    Q. Musculoskeletal
    R. Neurologic
    S. Endocrine
    T. Lymphatic

Objective Data

Vital Signs

1. Temp _____
2. Heart rate _____
3. Respiratory rate _____
4. Blood Pressure _____
5. Weight _____kg_____pounds _____ounces
6. Height _____cm_____inches
7. Body mass index _____
8. Parent–child interaction _____

General Appearance

1. Skin _____
2. Head _____
3. Face _____
4. Eyes _____
5. Ears _____
6. Nose _____
7. Mouth/throat _____
8. Neck _____
9. Thorax and lungs _____
10. Breast _____
11. Heart _____
12. Abdomen _____
13. Upper extremities _____
14. Lower extremities _____
15. Neurologic/reflexes _____
16. Genitalia _____
17. Rectum/anus _____
18. Results of laboratory tests _____

Assessment: _____

SAMPLE DOCUMENTATION: ADOLESCENT (AGES 12 YEARS AND OLDER)

Patient Name _____ Date of Birth _____
Source of Information _____ Relationship to Teen (mother, father, grandparent, caregiver)

Subjective Data

I. **Past Medical History**
II. **Past Surgical History**
III. **Family Medical History**
IV. **Immunization History**
V. **Allergies**
VI. **Injuries/Ingestions**
VII. **Emergency Room Visits**
VIII. **Current Medications**
IX. **Nutrition**
   A. **Typical Meals, and Snacks**
   B. **Amount of Juice/Soft Drinks/Fast Food Consumed Each Day**
   C. **Amount of Physical Activity/Screen Time Per Day**
X. **Elimination**
   A. **Constipation**
   B. **Diarrhea**
   C. **Binging**
   D. **Purging**
XI. **Safety**
   A. **Bicycle Helmet**
   B. **Stranger Safety**

      C. Seatbelts
      D. Dating Safety
      E. Bullying

XII. Sleep
      A. Hours of Sleep
      B. Bedtime

XIII. School Performance

XIV. BIHEADS Exam
      A. Body Image
      B. Home Environment
      C. Education (current educational level, achievement, plans for the future)
      D. Activities (friends, hobbies, interests)
      E. Drug Use
      F. Sexual Activity
      G. Suicidal Thoughts/Homicidal Thoughts or Fears

XV. Review of Systems
      A. General
      B. Integument
      C. Head
      D. Eyes
      E. Nose
      F. Ears
      G. Mouth
      H. Throat
      I. Neck
      J. Nodes
      K. Chest
      L. Respiratory
      M. Cardiovascular
      N. Gastrointestinal
      O. Genitourinary
      P. Gynecologic
      Q. Musculoskeletal
      R. Neurologic
      S. Endocrine
      T. Lymphatic

Objective Data

Vital Signs

1. Temp _____
2. Heart rate _____
3. Respiratory rate _____
4. Blood Pressure _____
5. Weight _____kg_____pounds _____ounces
6. Height _____cm_____inches
7. Body mass index _____
8. Parent–teen interaction _____

General Appearance

1. Skin _____
2. Head _____
3. Face _____
4. Eyes _____
5. Ears _____
6. Nose _____
7. Mouth/throat _____
8. Neck _____
9. Thorax and lungs _____
10. Breast _____
11. Heart _____
12. Abdomen _____
13. Upper extremities _____
14. Lower extremities _____
15. Neurologic/reflexes _____
16. Genitalia _____
17. Rectum/anus _____
18. Results of laboratory tests _____

Assessment: _____

Plan: _____

Answer Key to Review Questions

CHAPTER 1: CHILD HEALTH ASSESSMENT: AN OVERVIEW

1. a
2. d
3. b
4. a
5. c
6. a
7. b
8. a
9. b
10. b
11. a
12. a
13. d
14. a
15. c
16. b
17. d
18. a
19. b
20. c

CHAPTER 2: ASSESSMENT OF CHILD DEVELOPMENT AND BEHAVIOR

1. b
2. b
3. d
4. a
5. a
6. b
7. c
8. d
9. d
10. c
11. c
12. c
13. b
14. d
15. d
16. d
17. b
18. d
19. c
20. d

CHAPTER 3: COMMUNICATING WITH CHILDREN AND FAMILIES

1. a
2. c
3. b
4. c
5. a
6. c
7. a
8. c
9. d
10. a

CHAPTER 4: ASSESSMENT OF THE FAMILY

1. c
2. d
3. a
4. a
5. b

6. b
7. c
8. a
9. d
10. b

CHAPTER 5: CULTURAL ASSESSMENT OF CHILDREN AND FAMILIES

1. c
2. b
3. d
4. b
5. c
6. d
7. b
8. a
9. d
10. c

11. c
12. c
13. b
14. a
15. c
16. a
17. c
18. b
19. c
20. a

CHAPTER 6: OBTAINING THE PEDIATRIC HEALTH HISTORY

1. b
2. a
3. b
4. c
5. a
6. a
7. c
8. b

9. c
10. a
11. a
12. d
13. a
14. d
15. b

CHAPTER 7: ASSESSING SAFETY AND INJURY RISK IN CHILDREN

1. a
2. c
3. d
4. d
5. c
6. d
7. b
8. a
9. c
10. d

11. b
12. c
13. b
14. d
15. a
16. b
17. b
18. d
19. c
20. d

CHAPTER 8: THE PEDIATRIC PHYSICAL EXAMINATION

1. a
2. b

3. a
4. c

5.	b	13.	c
6.	b	14.	c
7.	d	15.	a
8.	b	16.	d
9.	b	17.	c
10.	a	18.	b
11.	d	19.	c
12.	c	20.	d

CHAPTER 9: THE HEALTH SUPERVISION VISIT: WELLNESS EXAMINATIONS IN CHILDREN

1.	b	11.	b
2.	c	12.	a
3.	c	13.	b
4.	c	14.	a
5.	a	15.	d
6.	c	16.	a
7.	b	17.	a
8.	d	18.	a
9.	c	19.	b
10.	d	20.	d

CHAPTER 10: ASSESSMENT OF NUTRITIONAL STATUS

1.	a	11.	c
2.	d	12.	a
3.	c	13.	b
4.	d	14.	a
5.	c	15.	d
6.	b	16.	c
7.	a	17.	d
8.	a	18.	b
9.	d	19.	a
10.	b	20.	c

CHAPTER 11: ASSESSMENT OF THE NEONATE

1.	a	11.	d
2.	b	12.	b
3.	d	13.	b
4.	a	14.	a
5.	a	15.	b
6.	c	16.	a
7.	c	17.	c
8.	d	18.	a
9.	b	19.	b
10.	a	20.	d

CHAPTER 12: ASSESSMENT OF THE INTEGUMENTARY SYSTEM

1. d		11. a	
2. b		12. d	
3. d		13. a	
4. d		14. b	
5. b		15. a	
6. c		16. c	
7. a		17. d	
8. d		18. a	
9. b		19. b	
10. c		20. d	

CHAPTER 13: ASSESSMENT OF THE HEAD, NECK, AND REGIONAL LYMPHATICS

1. d		11. a	
2. c		12. d	
3. a		13. c	
4. b		14. c	
5. c		15. b	
6. c		16. a	
7. c		17. a	
8. d		18. b	
9. b		19. c	
10. c		20. d	

CHAPTER 14: ASSESSMENT OF THE EARS

1. a		11. a	
2. d		12. c	
3. b		13. a	
4. c		14. c	
5. d		15. d	
6. b		16. d	
7. c		17. b	
8. b		18. b	
9. a		19. d	
10. c		20. a	

CHAPTER 15: ASSESSMENT OF THE EYES

1. d		7. c	
2. b		8. c	
3. a		9. d	
4. d		10. d	
5. b		11. c	
6. a		12. a	

13. d
14. c
15. a
16. a

17. c
18. b
19. c
20. a

CHAPTER 16: ASSESSMENT OF THE FACE, NOSE, AND ORAL CAVITY

1. a
2. b
3. a
4. a
5. b
6. b
7. c
8. b
9. d
10. a

11. b
12. a
13. c
14. a
15. b
16. b
17. c
18. b
19. a
20. d

CHAPTER 17: ASSESSMENT OF THE THORAX, LUNGS, AND REGIONAL LYMPHATICS

1. d
2. b
3. a
4. c
5. a
6. d
7. c
8. b
9. d
10. b

11. a
12. b
13. a
14. c
15. d
16. c
17. b
18. a
19. d
20. b

CHAPTER 18: ASSESSMENT OF THE CARDIOVASCULAR SYSTEM

1. b
2. a
3. c
4. a
5. c
6. a
7. b
8. d
9. d
10. a

11. a
12. b
13. b
14. a
15. a
16. d
17. b
18. d
19. a
20. b

CHAPTER 19: ASSESSMENT OF THE ABDOMEN AND REGIONAL LYMPHATICS

1. c
2. b
3. d
4. b
5. c
6. a
7. b
8. b
9. b
10. d

11. a
12. a
13. b
14. b
15. b
16. b
17. c
18. a
19. d
20. b

CHAPTER 20: ASSESSMENT OF THE REPRODUCTIVE AND GENITOURINARY SYSTEMS

1. b
2. a
3. b
4. c
5. b
6. d
7. c
8. a
9. b
10. b

11. b
12. a
13. d
14. d
15. a
16. d
17. b
18. a
19. c
20. b

CHAPTER 21: ASSESSMENT OF THE MUSCULOSKELETAL SYSTEM

1. a
2. c
3. b
4. a
5. a
6. a
7. d
8. b
9. b
10. b

11. a
12. b
13. c
14. b
15. a
16. b
17. a
18. c
19. b
20. d

CHAPTER 22: ASSESSMENT OF THE NEUROLOGIC SYSTEM

1. d
2. a
3. b
4. b
5. a
6. c
7. b

8. b
9. c
10. c
11. a
12. b
13. d
14. c

15. b		18. b	
16. b		19. c	
17. b		20. a	

CHAPTER 23: ASSESSMENT OF MENTAL DISORDERS IN CHILDREN AND ADOLESCENTS

1. d		11. d	
2. a		12. a	
3. c		13. c	
4. d		14. c	
5. c		15. b	
6. c		16. a	
7. b		17. d	
8. a		18. b	
9. d		19. c	
10. d		20. d	

CHAPTER 24: ASSESSMENT OF CHILD ABUSE AND NEGLECT

1. a		11. d	
2. d		12. d	
3. c		13. a	
4. a		14. d	
5. b		15. a	
6. a		16. d	
7. b		17. b	
8. a		18. a	
9. c		19. c	
10. b		20. a	

CHAPTER 25: THE COMPLETE HISTORY AND PHYSICAL EXAMINATION: FROM START TO FINISH

1. b		6. c	
2. a		7. b	
3. d		8. d	
4. b		9. c	
5. a		10. c	